THE ART OF SURRENDER

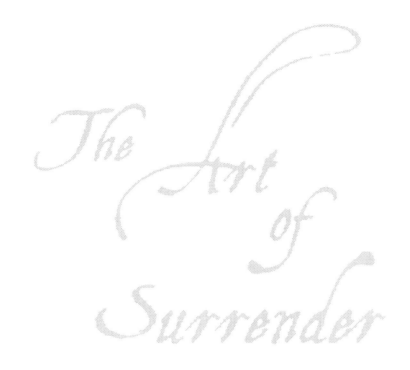

The Art of Surrender

BECCA SMITH

GLANCING ORPHEUS PRESS

ACORN BANK, MIDDLETOWN, CALIFORNIA

TO ORDER COPIES:

PAGE FREE PUBLISHING
Otsego, Michigan
www.pagefreeauthors.com
(866) 462-6657

Order through local, independent booksellers

ALSO AVAILABLE FROM:
alibris.com, amazon.com, barnesandnobel.com

ISBN: 1-58961-387-2

LIBRARY OF CONGRESS CONTROL NO:
2005905289

Contents

ART CREDITS

ALL ILLUSTRATIONS BY BECCA SMITH

This is a love letter written to my family and friends

Like Jonah

... The caretaker cottage in the vineyard stands nestled near the storage barn of Paraquat, Malathion and other common poisons, the spray rigs crawling the vineyard rows in every season. Born and raised in an agricultural region, I make light of exposure to commercial poisons, my body burden unappreciated until my momentous insight... The woman whose property I care for is recovering from breast cancer and dies of a reoccurrence ten years from now. Several women who work nearby have also been treated for the same disease.

During this time, I face that true love will not be easy as I imagined it. Instead I find love unexpectedly, in pleasure and rejection, intimacy and loneliness. I see that if my longtime love goes wrong, I will have nowhere to hide from the loss. I am a woman now, and childless. At thirty, I wonder how to create who I wish to be in the world.

I begin my story here, in my thirtieth year, with a puzzling message delivered in a dream about a whale. Misunderstood, a decade will pass before the message reveals its physical form. My life is a story unfolding as I wake from that dream, take pencil to paper and capture a mysterious communiqué, a poem in rhyme, "Discover the secret none can find." Words that fascinate, a story that survives over time, a tiny voice on a journal page, made mute by passing days until forgotten.

Oh mighty fish all black & shining
That rules my mind and leaves me pining
Grant A WISH or take me under
Lost to icy corridors of slumber
If you love me read my mind
Discover the secret none can find
If I wake and rise and if I sleep
I'll dream your restless turning in the deep.
A ship, a crew, a captain so handsome
All unknowing of my ransom
Whilst I like Jonah by fire and wit
Crowd the dark, the ETERNAL myth.
In the lighthouse glow a lonely swimmer
Looms up in the night a forgiven sinner
I go aground on that desolate beach
And the coal of myself is all that I keep.

I. WHEN THE BODY SPEAKS

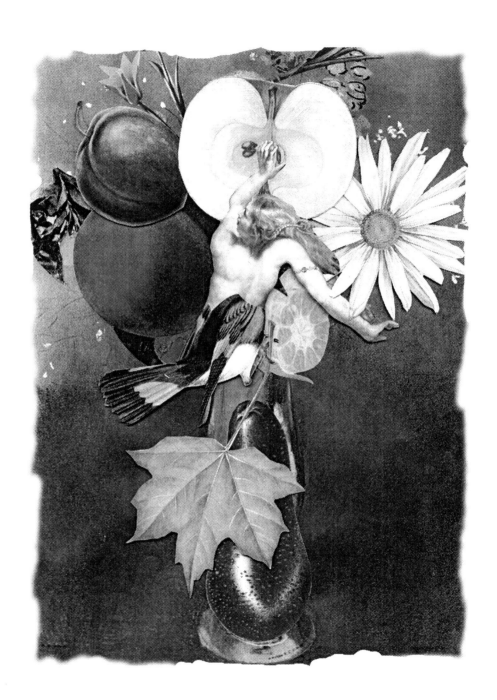

Think of losing your balance in a waist-high rapid. Without warning the colored stones under your feet are shifting, you are moving, all clever maneuvering and dignity lost, bashing your knees bloody on looming river rocks. Splashing, you flounder in a panic to the steep, tangled bank and claw your way into unfamiliar territory. Discovering a tumor grips the body with the same erosive force. You desperately try to keep pace with where your life is taking you.

Have you woken from sleep confused and failed to recognize everyday objects, the walls of your room or your own hand, strange on the ticking clock? Assimilating the implications of a tumor can be as disorienting. Alone, we enter a new reality where habitual assumptions have lost their power. The illusion of order fades to dark, overshadowed by the dawning realization of our own mortality.

I have so far escaped a further malignancy and these stories of my cancer layer like silt, geology of misfortune and redemption, perception and fact, medicine and superstition, dreams and visions, love and separation. Like Eve, I have learned much from a single bite, cast from ignorance into the world.

A DREAM...

on a warm *spring night, my brother and sister-in-law gather my family together. They explain that they are responsible for the soul of my friend and longtime muse, an artist. Unbeknownst to all of us, they are the guardians of her decayed body, which her soul still inhabits. They explain that several times a year they wash her in a ritual bath. This year they wish to enlist our help in this process.*

Crowding around a stone sarcophagus, we push back the heavy lid and gaze in. The artist's pearly skin is firm, muscular to the touch and the sacred positioning of her slender arms, archaic. But random areas of her flesh are fetid with old wounds, drawing the eye to areas of exposed bone on the chest and upper thigh. Her black hair, full and long, frames the shrunken skin on her mummified face. Here and there, brilliant white patches of skull appear.

Horrified, we look away. Someone vomits. We tip her out and into a burnished, antiquated metal tub, fashioned with ornate feet and embossed elements of sculpture. The water in the bath has a sumptuous quality, limpid and syrupy. Small flowers and herbaceous leaves float along the fragrant sur-face. She slips into this holy tincture and we dip our hands and wash her.

Amongst ourselves we repeatedly affirm that she is still living. We lift her from the water and onto a table. Her legs appear stronger. The taut skin covering her face is now serene and gleams with a gray iridescent polish. The mane of her hair is scattered with droplets of blue light.

We agree that the refreshed suppleness of her limbs lends permanence to her presence. Rolling her body on its side, my brother rests his fingers along her spine. Tilting his ear to her heart he says, "You see, you can hear her breathing. She's still breathing."

8

My companion of many years departed, mentoring and perceptions between us outgrown. My all-consuming business venture went wrong and was broken up and sold. After these simultaneous events, existential grief drained my life of meaning and I questioned my ability to love and be loved. Now, I work long hours to avoid lonely nights and am often exhausted. The increasingly listless energy of this new, solitary era troubles me but goes undiagnosed in body and spirit. A physical confirms my health, but I know I'm heartbroken and need reinventing. My dreams tell me so.

Like so many other days at work, I put aside my feeling of exhaustion for the demands of my job and my hope of inspiration. I haven't been sleeping well. I've recently taken to night sweats and strange dreams from which I wake frightened and confused. A mysterious and noxious onion odor periodically emitted by the first finger on my right hand is inexplicable, and it oddly shames me.

After a long afternoon of motivational meetings, I take a break to chat with women employees in my office. I'm making us all laugh by telling a joke. My gestures are exaggerated as I clown around. By chance, my right hand brushes the side of my breast. Through my bra and heavy denim shirt, I feel a hard area with the tips of my fingers. It's a shock that carbonates my blood.

I lose the momentum of the joke and feel the hard place again, deliberately this time. I say, "Oh my God, I feel a lump in my breast." The sudden quiet that descends on our group will be remembered for months afterward, privately worried on by each like a knife blade to

9

whetted stone. My spontaneous announcement embarrasses all of us. I dispel our awkwardness with a reassuring remark, go into the bathroom and feel the alien site again. I try desperately to remember if I've bumped my breast in some way, hit it with something, anything. The lump feels gigantic. I compare it in size to a large walnut. How have I not noticed it before? I tell myself, I'll think of it again when I get home.

At 8 PM, I walk into my kitchen like I would a boxing ring. There, anxiety has its way with me. All alone, I keep pressing on the hard spot in disbelief. I hang black crepe over the window of its reality. It catches and then falls, catches and falls.

I abandon the idea of dinner and go to bed. I lie on my side and feel my breast from that vantage point. As I do this, a realization stirs emotions quite removed from morbid paranoia. I know that in all the years of my breast exams, courageous handling or furtive groping, I've never felt anything like this. The edges are irregular; it's very hard and doesn't move. It hurts now that I've handled it so much. I take a deep breath and quiet my fingers.

As my tears come, I occupy parallel realities. I know that what I feel is a tumor but the knowledge keeps slipping away. My mind refuses to contain it. Why should I surrender to this new identity?

Nothing moves me to bargain with God. I rest my fingers on my breast again and caress the small, hard manifestation of my own mortality. I have never felt so alone. My bed, my body, the lamplight and my grief are all that is left of the world.

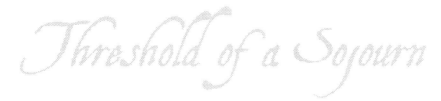

My doctor informs me that nothing has been detected on the mammography film. He's cheerful and expects we can clear the matter up, then and there. Over the course of two weeks, the hard place in my breast has mysteriously shrunk to half its original size. I tell him this change is easing my anxiety.

He examines me and then aspirates the lump with a needle in an attempt to draw liquid from what we hope is a cyst. Holding a dry syringe to the light, his mood changes to cautious concern. He recommends that we observe the lump over time for changes. He tells me he feels it would be safe to wait weeks or months, given my age, excellent health and unblemished mammogram. However, he tells me, if I would like to see a surgeon he will authorize it.

The nurse practitioner calls to congratulate me on a clear mammogram. I tell her that the lump hasn't proved to be a cyst. She pauses and then expresses concern, encouraging me to investigate further. I hang up the phone sick to my stomach. My back arches with the strength of my will. This cannot be happening. I call my doctor and discuss my desire to see a surgeon. I have just switched health insurance companies and I'm forced to delay making an appointment for nearly a month in order to guarantee coverage of what may come.

Hand of Faith

A period of suspension begins in which I live in fear. Time moves slowly. When I close my eyes I see myself from above, walking alone along an endless shoreline of the sea. I walk there, yet leave no prints, the only animate figure under a proximate sky.

To fight this fear, I have only my will and the bright banner of my pride, those two grand props now such false and useless attributes. I claim no bit of land, not even an oarless boat in which to rest. I know myself no more and only authenticity of being saves me from despair.

Hidden in the red cloak of my desperate desires, the voice of humility emerges to guide me. I have lived so long without faith; might I now call for hope as an abandoned child cries for food? Might I now realize a second chance to praise what has been given? Allow me to commit myself to hymns and scripts of tribute. A diary of starry nights filled with devotions carefully remembered at dawn.

Judge me not. Faith, you elusive charter, search for me within the Song of Solomon, as the lover seeks the Beloved in the garden of pomegranate trees.

II. A REIGN OF TRUTH

A Reign of Truth

I sit in the examination room on a padded table in a yellow paper gown. I'm still hoping for reprieve but the surgeon isn't talkative. Periodically he questions me while using his fingers like a pianist on a keyboard of breast flesh, ribs and hollows.

Twenty minutes go by. He washes his hands and clears his throat. He declares that were it not for supposed changes in the size of the lump, he would estimate that I have a 75 percent chance of having breast cancer. He reveals that he has also detected a small mass in the pit of my arm.

We schedule a surgical biopsy to take place in two days. As he and his nurse and I sit in front of the scheduling book, I immediately sense the intimacy that compassion brings. I perceive the gravity of my situation in the urgency with which he includes me in the arrangement of his schedule. The surgeon and the nurse relate to me with a fraternal quality, and my surface compliance feels symbolic. I see the two of them as my ushers to a newly found world. They view me as a person yet in the dark and shine what lights they have to guide me. These medical formalities allow me an initiation period. They give me time to

I tell myself, hush your mind. What's happening inside you? It's as though I've taken a draught of heated and honeyed liquid. It saturates every cell and divides my very self in two. From one part, a soundless howling rises. A gale wind, stripping away all thought like leaves from wood. I want to strike the surgeon, leap on his shoulders and break his neck with my thighs. Kill the messenger or make him call out and weep with me. My other self captures and herds this rage, wakened as it has from the anxious expectation of decades. I see a graphic image of my own mother's scarred chest. My face flushes a deep rose. I'm steady, friendly and direct. I question the surgeon closely. I keep pace with this cool, composed man who acquaints me with the prospect of death. I'm not letting his beliefs inside my body. Can I still claim a contrary fate?

assimilate the potentialities, struggle with the terrible erosion of reality I feel activated by the possibility of death. As we speak together calmly, a fierce and primal part of me grips a superior hope.

My mother is waiting for me in the lobby. She searches my face as I come through the office door, so alert and brave. I want only to comfort her, smile and give good news. Instead I take her arm and force a trembling to vacate my face. On hearing my report, her body momentarily sags with the burden of content. She straightens her shoulders and pats my arm.

Our silence begs the question, how far are we still from the bottom? We walk through the surgeons' lobby in the weighty air of suspended time, slow-motion turning for one last look at the past. My mother, how will she privately endure this? She does not ask me WHY out loud. She already knows this does not matter.

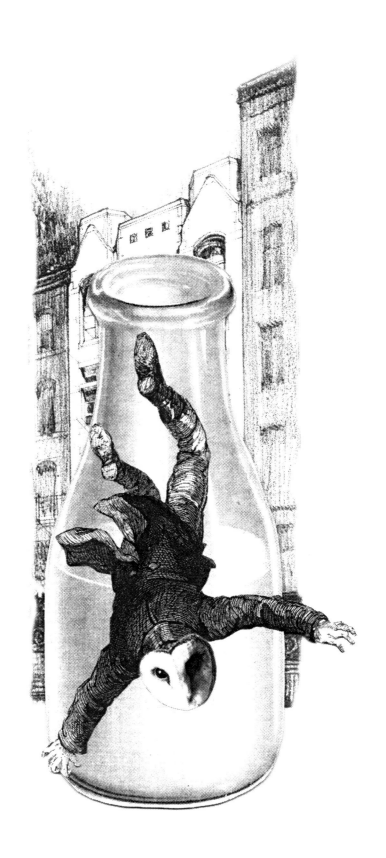

In the operating room, I drift up through the levels of anesthesia. Slurring my words, I report to the handsome anesthesiologist that I have been at the beach in my dream. He laughs. My first thought of consciousness is to appease them.

My surgeon is still sewing up my breast. I can sense the tugging of his tools in my deadened flesh. Struggling inside the veil of a drugged sleep, I strain to decipher the tenor of his voice for a clue to my dawning fate. When he comments to the nurse that my tissue has been a long time at the lab, my heart drops like an anchor in bottomless water. He leaves my side and crosses the room. He places a call. In the indelible voice of professionalism, I hear him say, "I see, uh-huh." He comes back to my side and leans down. Through his mask he says, "I'm sorry, but you have cancer."

He exits the refrigerated operating room as I begin to sob. A nurse holds my hand and tells me that she has survived breast cancer and is doing well. The jolly orderly brings me Kleenex. No one wants to see me cry for long. They do their best to comfort me for a few awkward minutes, after which I will never see them again.

Alone in the recovery room, I feel so strange, as though I've been abducted. I cannot connect to the woman I have been. I'm thrown overboard and survive the open maw of the waves. There I am washed clean of all pretense and false hope. My mother and older brothers rush in. They stand, courageous, rehearsed, at the foot of my bed. They all speak at once in practiced assurances. Fear moves loose in the room.

The surgeon enters and shakes their hands and articulates my options in a concise voice and measured tone. We ask questions which he answers with respect for our perceptions. He provides us with statistical data and his recommendations. I decide without hesitation on a lumpectomy and the removal, if necessary, of my lymph nodes. The surgery will be performed in two days. Afterward, I think of the surgeon. He, perhaps more than anyone, understands the dire possibilities in my future. Yet I refuse to embrace his prophecies of chemotherapy and autologous bone marrow transplants. I know he hopes that I will meet what lies ahead with courage and intelligence. But I dream of a simple pathology, one where I can heal my body, not "treat" it.

I lie unmoving and exhausted, angry at my body's betrayal. I tell myself that my goodness or righteousness will save me from further betrayals. This tumor is a terrible mistake. A celestial hand will switch the lab files. A hospital administrator will call with an apology in the morning.

Two days later, I lie on a gurney again. I'm still attempting to change my reality. I hear no music inside me. If I allowed it, could I die like a fawn of fear and frozen trembling? In my mind there are brief prayers from an undiscovered source, rationalizations in a tolerant voice. "I've been kind and thoughtful to others. I've done nothing wrong. Spare me death."

I have trust in my surgeon. I want him to believe that the harmful tumor is well contained. I smile and speak politely with everyone. Like Alice in Wonderland, I've stood up, cool and composed, from my long fall to this other world. I tell myself that nothing, no madness, no horror, will surprise me. I am practicing curiosity. I will praise what is overwhelming.

I'm silenced with drugs. Then waking surrounded by family, gazing at me with concern and tenderness. They take turns sitting in the chair next to my bed, assuring me with their love. Several friends come and go, consulting with family members in the hallway. The drugs I've been given dull the discomfort of the wounds and drain in my side. A landscape of pain has been reduced to the peculiar ridged sensation of trauma and flesh more dead than alive. I communicate from behind the barricade of my altered senses.

My surgeon comes in for a consultation. He refrains from saying too much. He feels the surgery has gone very well. He is sure that he has been able to remove all of the affected tissues. However, we must wait several days for the results of the pathology test of the lymph nodes he has removed. He announces that he has seen fit to remove twenty-three of the nodes in my right arm. Every one he can find. I have recently versed myself in cancer pathology, yet I choose to ignore the implication of the removal of so many lymph nodes.

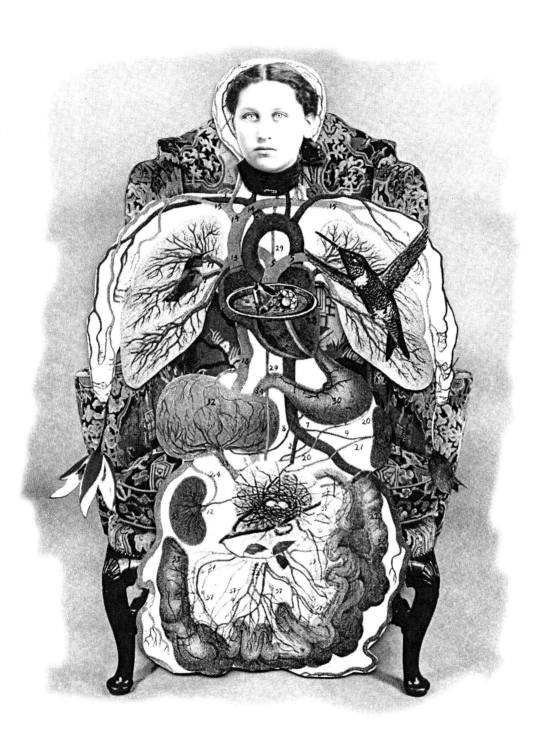

I'm trying to dress myself in my mother's bathroom, but every movement brings acute pain and tears. Traveling between the hospital and the house, the pain medication has worn thin. I look at my face and chest in the mirror and for the first time I see the chemotherapy port embedded in my chest. My imagination grasps the actuality of the chemotherapy drugs in my future.

My breast and side are heavily bandaged, but the chemo port stands out in a proclamation of events beyond my control. I break down in a rage of tears. My mother begins to bend over and sob. I can't cope with her grief and mine as well, so I yell obscenities and curse the doctors to chill our emotions. I shout out in anger at this terrible invasion, this impermissible, plastic deed. "Those sons of bitches. Fuck them. What do they know? I won't do it. No one can make me. Damn it. Shit, it's so ugly. Oh God, Mom, what will happen to me? My arm, it hurts. It hurts." I haven't understood what my casual consent of the chemo port would mean. I've prayed not to wake up with one. This insidious disk of polymer bulging beneath my skin represents an assumption of a serious pathology and the finality of chemotherapy. I'm not ready to decipher the implications of its presence.

My father drops by for a visit at my mother's house. I cry and hold my face in my hands when I see him. I tell him, "Dad, I'm so afraid." He kneels by my chair and leans his face against me. "You'll be OK."

I eat dinner with my parents. It's the first time I've been alone with the two of them since they took me to dinner on my twenty-first birthday, nineteen years ago. They are divorced and very rarely together in the same place. It's a revelation to study the old habits of their familial bond. We laugh together at each one's version of the same events. They tell me the well-loved family stories of their courtship and early married life. They review the history of their youth together growing up in Napa Valley in the thirties, World War II, Greenwich Village after the war and their dream of artistic fame. They tell me the story of my birth, each one adding a detail here and there. A mood comes over me, a powerful tug to my genetic chain. I had forgotten the sensation I relive in their presence. For a keen moment, I am just a child with her parents, physically belonging to them again. I relish, objectively, this richness I come from. I feel a renewed gratefulness in their company and it moves me to a profound realization.

I've struggled through the diagnosis and surgery with the notion of being punished by God or fingered by the universe. Despite my intellectual understanding of cancer, I've experimented with the idea of sacrificed health as punishment for my failure to appreciate the gift of creativity in my life. I've ignored and abandoned my bliss and blame myself for this disease. Amidst my parents' laughter and poignant remarks, I begin to perceive the real meaning I will make of this illness. Could it be a gift? Dimly, it comes to me that this cancer has nothing to do with sacrifice. Instead, I will be shown a way to change my life and leave old grief behind. I will be asked to accept more love, more unconditional gifts of expression, a life more attuned to the receptive spirit, however short.

My parents have filled me up, helped me know who I am again. Their steady company balances the morning's terrifying view of my bandages and chemo port. With my mind's eye, I clasp my parents to my heart, like treasure filling the gouges of a ravaged chest.

A Blight of Nodes

The eternity of five days is relinquished to the past. My surgeon removes my bandages and painfully slides the drain from my side. I see my first view of the maiming, long, reddened incisions that run under my arm and across the side of my breast. He chastises me for being unable to lift my arm over my head. My face burns. I don't complain about how I've wept from pain practicing the recommended exercises without the aide of physical therapists. He tells me, "You've got to get tough, kid."

I don't comprehend his discourse on my future and keep silent my resentment. I'm wary of this man who put the chemo port in my chest. He describes how many tendons it was necessary to cut in order to remove my lymph nodes. "Regrettably," he remarks, "you may suffer chronic pain beneath your right shoulder blade." What can I say in answer, thank you? I want to lash out at him, be cynical, but his mood frightens me. There is a remote quality to his body language. My ego wrings its hands and chirps, "Keep on his good side; it will affect what he has to say." He leaves me and I dress.

My mother and brother return with him for our consultation. He tells us that ten out of twenty-three nodes in my arm revealed evidence of cancer. For the second time, he stresses the topic of autologous bone marrow transplant and recommends an oncologist. At this news, my brother turns to stone, and my mother grips his arm. They dredge up questions and speak in stifled tones of shock and defeat. I've been reading up on breast cancer and the shortened life spans of women with nodal involvement. Chemotherapy is recommended with any sign of cancer in the nodes. A count of ten nodes is considered high

risk for recurrence and death. The possibility of cancer cells having entered my bloodstream is likely. The potential for microscopic bits of cancer having lodged in my lung, liver, brain, or bones is a reality I must now face.

As the surgeon's voice fades into the background, I nod in blank acknowledgement. Now I understand his mood and regrets for me. The skin on my face begins to crawl and sweat and my stomach is a swamp of fluid. Notions of my life are devastated by his words, ambition felled like a sudden clear cut, a pile of scrapped lumber ready for burning.

Sitting here on the examining table, my spirit removes itself from present company. I crave a rocky outcrop and the blue roof of heaven, a silent place of austere solitude for the privacy of a savage weeping. I know the sound of this humid rage, its rhythm and vibration, my bloody fists, will bring no shame. I've read that human tears are music to the Gods.

Oncology

I'm learning to proclaim what I am willing to risk. I want a physician who respects me, one I can trust. I want a doctor who believes, passionately, in what is to be done, but one who can still listen. I want a marriage of true minds, a person who inspires my affection. I am so lucky to find him.

My siblings, my mother and I gather together in a small examining room. Each of us has arrived prepared with our separate questions. My oncologist, the first of three I plan to interview, enters the room. He's a young man, younger than I. He is handsome and energetic in a blue striped shirt. A stethoscope rests around the back of his neck. I see him rise mentally to the unusual occasion of so many family members.

He shakes hands and introduces himself to everyone in the room. He sits on a swivel chair and reads my pathology report aloud. He makes his recommendation plain. He explains the concept of what he names a stem-cell rescue, this term being synonymous with autologous bone marrow transplant. He further explains that I fit a profile that makes me a candidate for this cutting-edge experimental treatment.

I fit the research trial specifications for a number of reasons. We must assume, from the presence of cancer in my lymph nodes, that cancerous cells have invaded my blood. Before I would be considered a true candidate, I'm to be thoroughly tested for the presence of metastasized cancer in my organs and bones. My tumor is non-hormonally related, which is considered more serious since the estrogen-inhibiting drug Tamoxifen will be less effective. Since I'm only forty and in excellent health, and my tumor was small and smooth around the edges, it is expected that I would respond well and better resist the ill effects of a rigorous course of treatment such as stem-cell rescue.

My oncologist lays out his plan. My treatment will first involve a course of high-dose chemotherapy, a single dose each twenty-one days, a total of four doses in all. The harvest of my stem cells (new-born cells produced by my bone marrow) and their analysis and cleaning would be the next procedure. Then, if I choose, I will undergo the transplant as an outpatient or in a hospital. There I will receive radically concentrated doses of chemotherapy to kill my exist-ing bone marrow. My previously harvested, now purified stem cells will then be reintroduced into my bloodstream, where they will, it is hoped, find their way back to my bone marrow. This treatment will be enacted in isolation, as I will endure a period of time without immunity. If the stem cells fail to engraft, my immune system will be beyond repair. The third stage of treatment involves six weeks of radiation.

I look at my oncologist and consider his trust worth. He's so young. How can he face people, day after day, with their worst fears? I'm astonished at his level of fresh energy, his willingness to engage and his capacity for eye contact and humor. I realize that it is his job to sell me on the idea of the treatments but, despite his pitch, I detect no arrogance.

I know that he understood immediately that he is dealing with an informed patient, one who could decide against chemotherapy based on real research. Our questions and answers to each other define our belief systems. He believes a stem-cell transplant is the best possible cure, and I see that his sincerity of feeling and commitment to chemotherapy is genuine.

He looks directly at me and explains that he expects my decision-making process will be difficult and complex. He suggests that he arrange for me to speak to several of his patients, women who have undergone the stem-cell process. He tells us that his most recently recovered patient is planning to be married in several months.

I say had he mentioned that a good marriage rounded out the treatment, persuasion would have been unnecessary. My humor both surprises and relieves him. We all laugh. Already, I want this man to believe I will get well. I know that I can be myself with him; his integrity is obvious and because of this, a small part of me willingly acquiesces to the consideration of his plan.

His nurse takes me aside and leads me into the chemotherapy treatment area. He shows me a chemo port and I see for the first time the object onto which I have focused my fear. He shows me how the nurses will access my veins through the opening in the plastic disk. He explains that should I decide on the transplant, yet another port will be implanted in the other side of my chest.

I hyperventilate as I study the color snapshots of transplant patients pinned on a corkboard, the chronological record of their journey to a chemical hell. The courage and humor in the gaunt and wasted faces touch me like a hundred ghostly hands, a force of feathers, shepherding me where I do not wish to go. Only the calm and kindly spirit of the male nurse keeps me from bolting through the door.

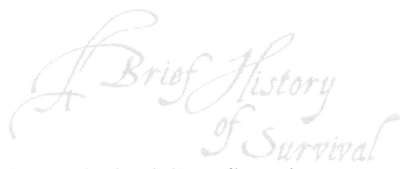

A Brief History of Survival

I question my mother about the history of her own breast cancer. She is seventy-two years old. I've never asked her before to tell me the entire story without stopping. "You were four and I was thirty-six. In 1958, two years after the birth of the youngest of you, I thought that the hard place in my breast should be looked into..."

She tells me that after exploratory surgery, in an abrupt and brutal manner, she awoke having had a radical mastectomy, with its accompanying disfiguring scar. In those days, a hysterectomy was automatically performed. The terrifying lead blanket and the peering faces of nurses through the tiny window of the radiation room are her most vivid recollections. She only mentions the result: terrible burns on the scarred tissue left to hug the contours of her rib cage.

My mother assures me that she willed herself through the experience and the fear of reoccurrence by praying that she remain alive to raise her five children. Each time the fear of a tumor rose up in her, she would immediately and harshly banish it, a technique I decide to adhere to. My mother asks me whether or not I remember her time in the hospital. She has never asked me this before.

I close my eyes and see three stills in faded colors. I was already six the first time I saw her scar.

I open the bathroom door to see
you emerging through the steam from the
shower. I look up and see where your breast has been.
You deftly move your towel to cover the profound emptiness
of twisted lavender skin. The beauty of your single breast is not
enough to wrench my gaze from a remaining glimpse of carved skin at
the top of your shoulder. But you dazzle me, shape-shift, Aphrodite
brushing her hair before my eyes. I learn nothing
of the pity of scars from you.

In a space of bright light, a willowy woman holds me in the stairwell. My small
arms are pale against her charcoal neck. Home from the operation, my mother
cannot lift me. Nor can she lift the baby. I am in the care of this woman, come
from the church to help. She is my private delight. We have a joke. This is how
she entices me to speak. Otherwise, I am silent.

She asks me, "What you want for lunch?"

"Tuna."

"Tuna! Girl, all you ever want is tuna. You're
my tuna girl." It is her laugh that I
am waiting for.

A
wild head thrown back laughter,
shaking, my body rising and falling in her large
embrace, a contagious laughter that swells up the stairs
and into the hall, a laugh whose joy I command and herd,
room to room, to find and kindle my mother.

Lastly, I see the heavy furniture and dim corners of my Aunt Margie's house.
Why did they leave us here, and what is The Hospital? I come out of the bath-
room and Margie is there. She asks, "Was it number one or number two, dear?"
Her question fills me with anxiety. Why does she want to know this? At our house,
we use the real names of body functions. I'm silent. I want to be good, go back home,
where everything will be the same again.

Is number one or two a reference to the bowel? I have no idea. Since "two" implies
a weightier matter I announce, "number one," and am instantly seized with a
paroxysm of guilt for having lied. The appearance of purity must now suffice. I
retreat to my secret place in the hollow under the cedar trees but do not stay.
It has never felt ominous before now.

III. PRAISING

.

Cure by Poison

TALES OF THE FIRST CHEMO

I nourish an active hatred for my chemotherapy port, a corporate polymer prop lodged beneath my freshly scarred skin. I harbor morbid fears of terminal infections caused by incorrect flushing or unclean manipulation of the plastic disk. Perhaps I've read too many manuals. I want to viciously slap the face of any person telling me to think of chemo poisons as "rainbow juice." As I wait for my first treatment to begin, the attendant adjusts the bags of colored fluids. Fear breeds itself in my expectation of the unknown. I ask myself, what will I sacrifice to this? What can I understand and learn from this poisonous permeation?

The nurse swabs my chest with brackish iodine anesthetic. Skillfully, she pushes the blunt needle, like a thickened thumbtack, through the flesh of my chest and into the opening of the port. I gasp and hold my breath. I have a dread of needles. My body is very sensitive to medications and the first dose of anti-nausea drugs sickens me with a lurid high. It's with great effort that I keep my eyes open and chin up, trying to ignore a case of mild tunnel vision. Next the nurse hangs the first bag of chemo drugs to my IV stand. Drip by drip, it enters my bloodstream. Down the tube and through the port, the blue fluid runs cold in my veins.

The nurses watch me closely, see how anxious I am and offer me a blanket. My oncologist arrives to check my vital signs and

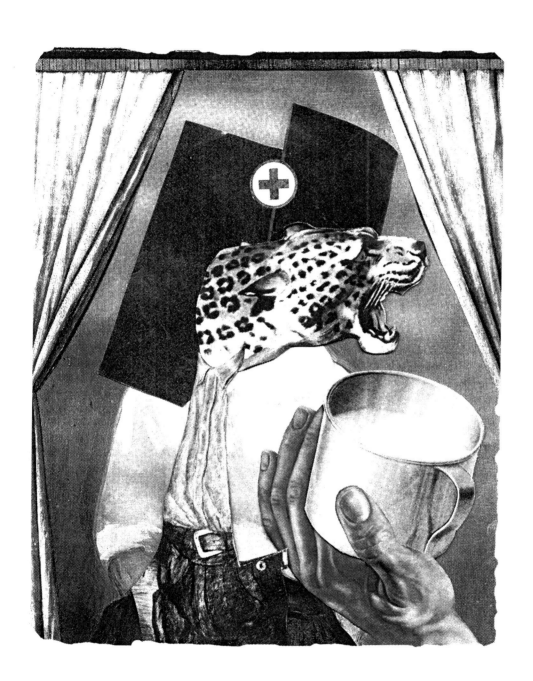

encourage me. As I lift my head to greet him, the room spins and my fingers fail to connect with his outstretched hand. My head gives a dopey swing. He squats by my chair, touches my arm with kindness, but the reality of the room seems very narrow, no escaping the truth of a tumor. The agony of my surrender is more difficult than the discomfort of any medicine. My life has led me to a meager pride. There is a shame inherent to chemotherapy, as though to say, no one with any self-esteem would permit this fouling of the body.

Who but I will honor so private a passage? I ask myself, where are my dancing maidens and the virgin prince? Where are the wise women and medicine men, sprinkling me with gold pollen? Is this attentive nurse my Ceberus, the drugs my water of forgetfulness? Is my young oncologist the boatman who rows me across?

I close my eyes to see the red tube of my vein and then move along the subclavian wall with the stream of toxic fluids. Stroking the broad tributary, I listen to the creaking oar-locks and lean to accept the mysteries of that near, distant and elemental shore.

I am remembering how to pray.

I recall a morning in my seventh year, walking alone to St. John's church, relishing the privacy of a holy and solitary moment. In my Sunday best, I carry my small prayer book in a special way. I mimic the biblical story of the boy who hid the holy sacrament inside his robe. It was his mission to deliver the consecrated bread into the hands of secret worshippers. In the catechism illustration I've studied, he holds the sacrament to his chest, protecting it just so. This thin bread is a fragile metaphor, sacred and surrounded with bright flames. He carries the host as though it were the still-beating heart of Jesus. The caption describes how the boy is discovered and brutalized by Roman soldiers. No matter: in the hands of brutes, his face in the picture reveals only the private bliss of divinity. As I walk, I hold my Sunday missal to my own heart, head down, inspired and alone. Lost in child-like thoughts of suffering and goodness, an overwhelming influence of love envelops me. In the presence of this love, I am aware of a deep yearning and joy alive in the world. No explanation of its power is necessary. With my child's reverence, I join in the solace of that exquisite yearning; I know that I belong there.

Now, I wish to locate the comfort of this presence. For thirty years, beauty and nature have triggered longing, but never a prayer. I've struggled with a memory of divinity like an interrupted dream one cannot recapture. The divorce of my parents nurtured a cynical view of all religious impulses. After that betrayal, God was a statue, burdenbent at the knees, his epitaph reading, "Broken Promise."

39

Thinking I may die, I feel change flood over me. I'm caught up in an overwhelming desire to praise. I realize that I've suppressed a grand passion for gratitude and creative solitude. I realize that I've never appreciated my roots in the drama and majesty of ritual, the mysterious Latin mass, hymns, incense and robes woven through the sensory life of my childhood. Alone in my bed at night, I attempt to sort out a symbolic face or voice of consciousness to embrace. I don't question my need for a protector or figure of love for me to shower my affection. I hunger not for doctrine but for a lover of my spirit. My desires are simple. Left alone, I praise the delirious preciousness of each moment and choose the Virgin of Guadalupe to love.

I

A year and half ago I broke with my companion of sixteen years. We have had less and less contact. He reemerges now from his new relationship, offering to help me build a shrine against a high wall in my garden. Together we sculpt it with chicken wire and cover it with a coating of concrete. I paint its surface and decorate the gray brick behind it with Guadalupe's flaming aura: burnt orange, turquoise and gold. Inspired by the tradition of Mary vision stories, we build her a place of worship. Nasturtiums will climb its sides and flower.

He has brought a gift of yellow roses. I plant them for adornment at the base of the shrine. In the middle of the structure we've carved an alcove three feet in height. Its arched stucco ceiling is painted blue

It's late and I'm awake
in my bed, restless and fearful of sleep. I
pray to Guadalupe for comfort. I lie with my eyes closed
in meditation and release a sensation of grief tightening my chest.
Several minutes go by. Spontaneously, my mind is filled with the image of two enormous, dusty brown feet. They stand an inch from the surface of my chest. Behind them
is the icon of Guadalupe's crescent moon embraced by an angel.
In a panic I think if she stands on me, she'll crush me with her weight. We exchange
silent thoughts: "I'm afraid," "Don't fear me." She pivots herself forward, to hover
facedown the full length of my body. Her face, an inch from mine, exhales a
Madonna's intimate breath. Her belly and breasts hang down inside her robes and
brush me. She hesitates. It makes it so real. Then the vision of her sinks into my
body. A brief image of her blue veil, covered in stars, floats, transparent
just beneath the surface of my skin. I open my eyes, close
them, and drop off into sleep.

and
decorated
with thin gold stars.
The inner ledge of the alcove holds a large dish of water. It makes a tiny pond for bees and songbirds.

Tonight, I feel well enough to float flowers on its surface and light candles and incense around its rim. I sit in the cricket-broken silence of the summer evening and watch slender curls of scented smoke rising. I think about love. Lights play on the water, reflected through the colored glass of the votive candles, ruby red, indigo and green. I'm recovering physically and emotionally from my first chemotherapy treatment. I haven't slept well in days.

...sleeping, i dream *that my mother and I, and my dog Josephine, are alone together on the banks of a wide, slow-moving river. The morning weather is sunny with a fresh breeze. The water smells of clean mud and young fish.*

The dog and I are working in the shallows and my mother lies above us on top of a high grassy bank. A beautiful and youthful presence, she wears a white lace dress and sash. Her body lies nested in grass, propped on one elbow. She calls out to me with her concerns: what about my work responsibilities, my safety, and the safety of the dog? She mentions the soon-to-be-spoiled lunch that should be eaten. Her brow is furrowed with unnecessary worry.

I am in the river, thigh-deep. A swarm of tiny colored butterflies are blown about, out above the middle current. I'm dressed impeccably in waders, wool pants, and a watermelon-colored gabardine shirt. My hair is flowing long and the sun sparkles red in its light. At ease with myself, I'm the picture of health. My sleeves are rolled up high. I can see my arm muscles pumping. My hands are covered in wet, brown river mud.

I'm working with intense concentration and a long iron pole on a log-jam of giant trees. The tangle is very complex; I face a massive puzzle of exposed roots twenty to thirty feet in diameter. Mighty trunks steam in the crispness of the morning air. I'm using all of my powers, physical and intellectual, to position every move of the iron pole. Each time I succeed in dislodging a tree trunk and it slides and crashes into the current, I feel more confident. They are so beautiful, the vision of them, their breathlike steaming and the weightless grace of their floating downriver.

The dog is happy too. She lifts her head and strains her wilder senses, deciphering messages on the air. We stand together, one protecting the others' peace. Dragonflies and kingfishers dart and weave in choreographed motions around us.

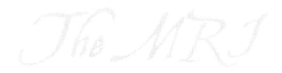

I

I'm breathless and anxious as I lie in the dark under a machine that scans my bones for odd bits of malignancies. I stare at the electronic image of my body on a television screen and will health into the image of my marrow. I wish the technician would describe what she is seeing. I understand all the reasons against giving partial or premature information to patients. Still, I want the facts as they happen.

I'm tested to passively reveal myself to an outsider's scrutiny and influence, willingly allow the study of my bones and blood. Suddenly, I'm to believe that my life is in their hands. I succumb, warily, to their expertise. See there, a person unknown to me reads the story of my bones, snaps a quick photo of my heart to file. Here, this stranger cuts me open and peers inside, manipulates my organs and tissue while I lie powerless in sleep. They wash my blood from their hands. Perhaps, consciously or unconsciously, without my permission, they look for evidence of my soul spirit. Finding no proof, they return to a belief in the omnipotent power and importance of medical intervention.

You might ask how I can be anything but grateful for technology? Yet, after being sewn up or sent away, it is difficult to integrate these acts, akin as they are to loveless sex, crucial moments between strangers. The poking and prodding, and the questionnaires I endure, are exhausting. I have to struggle against the residual emotions of invasion and generate an awkward sense of gratitude. I convince myself to claim these procedures as my own procreative acts and create spontaneous rituals around them.

I arrive for my MRI. Magnetic resonance imaging is standard procedure for those whose pathology raises suspicions of tumors that have metastasized. The technician will be looking for cancer in the tissue under my skull. Actually, I'm elated over the prospect of seeing pictures of my brain, but my inspiration fails me when they leave me inside the machine.

I'm completely surrounded as I lie on my back with a few inches of space between my face and the hard surface of the tube. They've given me headphones and a choice of tapes to disguise the thunderous transmission of sound waves. The kindly woman technician sits in an outer room and communicates with me through my headset. She reassures me, and offers a tranquilizer should I need it.

II

To drown out the noise, I listen to a tape entitled *Sounds of the Sea*, but the free and lonely rhythm of breaking waves opens my grief and fear. Tears roll down my neck. I call out in my mind to Guadalupe. I ask her again, "Please, Mother, help me now."

She enters my imagination young, brown and beautiful, barefoot, in her signature blue robe embroidered with gold stars. I see our distant figures on a third-world beach, overcast, with bleak palms and muggy air. The pounding sounds of the MRI become jackhammers from a distant building project. I see a rough, windy stretch of sand and unfinished architecture against a leaden sky.

We walk, arm in arm, laughing like girls. She sits in the sand and I dance for her in the wave foam, slowly, with feeling. She gazes at me encouragingly, as though I were her first-born daughter smiling back at her from my crib. I come to her, lay my head in her lap and she rocks me in her arms. I study her face, her single earring, and her lips. Her teeth flash white when she smiles. Her jeweled hands brush my face like the wings of a delicate bird. She sings a low melody and dries my tears with an edge of silk.

The technician's voice through the headphones interrupts my vision. She tells me that my hour is nearly complete. Turning inward again to my private mind, Guadalupe, her hands outstretched with love, glides in reverse away from me down the beach.

The technician risks telling me that the pictures look good. I sit with her in front of a large console screen filled with photographic images. In the frames of the negatives, I see an outline of my skull enclosing the curly texture of my brain. The mystery of the tissue I witness thrills me. My eyes move to the familiar outline of my facial features, photographed minutes before. They are soft and sweet, holding an expression of gentleness and serenity.

In the glare of the changing room light, I bow my head in gratitude against the wall. I put my fingers to my face and lips, as though to memorize the touch of a love supreme.

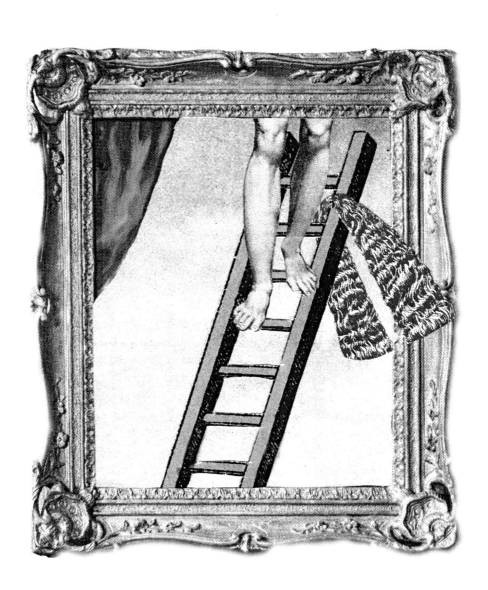

Reverse Rapunzel

For Patty Sue

My hair is falling out. This means I'm dying. The skin on my scalp is no longer alive. The root of each hair stands akimbo, singed and brittle in its dead pore. No more little lights shine or sparkle on its surface. My friend shears my hair in stages. I hold my severed braid like a beautiful trout, gasping in the air around my hands. The red lights are the first lights to go.

My pillow in the morning, a loose nest built of locks and strands. Thin piles of hair cover the papers on my desk. At the sight of them I think, "Hiroshima, Hiroshima, Hiroshima." After showering, the hair on my body is lost to the friction of toweling, my Venus mound suddenly exposed and disturbingly unfamiliar.

Alone, I gaze at my face in the mirror. My skin glistens an unearthly opaque. The hair I have left perches painfully on my scalp. I kneel in the bath and put my head near the spout. I wash away that hair, dead grass, with handfuls of warm water.

I clasp my bald head with a midwife's grip. I'm reborn bereft of vanity. My scalp is free of the sting and burn. I'm goofy and short of breath. Left here and there, thin strands I twirl the feathers of the strangest bird. The shape of my head is becoming. No wig-shop masquerade can persuade me. I desire the truth of this telling beauty and anoint my pate with oil.

49

The path below my house winds through a meadow to my friend's cottage. I follow its steep slope into her enthusiastic and loving embrace. She studies my new hairless look and we laugh together, discussing the shape of my head and the fashion merits of bald and straggly. Michael waits inside and the three of us try on Jeani's collection of funny hats, vintage, wacky and weird. My appearance doesn't shock them and we celebrate my transition without hesitation. With best friends, humor over my situation is a ready antidote to overwhelming change. They pass off baldness as "exciting travel to new identities."

My friends show me the way to survive my losses by never taking ourselves too seriously. All loss is relative. As an example, Michael reaches into the hatbox and grabs a pair of pointy, vintage eyeglasses and a powder blue forties church hat, his frizzy hair sticking from underneath it, down his neck to his shoulders. He stands and begins to toddle around the living room in a perfect imitation of a bow-legged old lady. We laugh until we cry, happy to be living, still within reach of each other.

Visiting with Angels

do i find *the approach of death erotic? Is eroticism the flower-draped con-cubine of suffering? As my spirit wakens, its vitality sweeps through me like a burst of blossoms. I'm the descendant of women who covered their heads before entering church, honoring the old idea that women's hair aroused the lust of angels. Scarred and bald, am I still beautiful?*

In a dream…I live, holed up, in a seedy apartment building. As I walk the hallways, they sway and heave like endless corridors on a passenger train. In the dim, oily light, the walls throb to the tempo of anonymous dramas behind each closed door. The hallway rug makes a polluted bed for the disenfranchised. Their periodic outbursts mingle with distant shouting and the sobbing of infants in a general and anguished fugue.

I am at home here and cheerfully greet people by name. My legs are long. Approaching a stranger, handsome and inviting, I do a mambo walk with my skirt above my hips. Smiling, we take our pleasure pressed against the green and waxy wall.

I enter my room and sit down backwards in a chair. I put my face inside a glassless window in the wall. Facing me through the window is a large, dark-skinned man. He's seated on a chair, in a room, on the opposite side of the wall. Breathing, our faces barely touch.

We begin to speak of love in a musical language of eternal murmurs, passionate and sweet, our hands braced at the sill. His face is beaded in sweat, which trickles in rivulets down the contours of his powerful chest. Truly, madly, deeply, these words of love caress me, the sensual yearning so profound the soul cannot witness it and causes the eyes to flutter and close.

THE SORROWS OF
THE SECOND CHEMO

With the second treatment of chemotherapy, I wade deeper and deeper into the realm of unknown futures. I do not know how to prepare for an early death, only how to accept what is. Accept each moment, soberly and with the greatest measure of grace I can assume.

A voice is with me now, a stowaway that emerges in dreams. A friend's voice that whispers, "surrender," gently lifting grief like a mirror to my face. I know I'm filled with a wry, overripe sadness. I try to let it go. A sense of acceptance takes up residence in my heart, accompanied by the melancholy jingle of some small, bright coins of self-compassion. Their tinkling music, fragments of love song sewn in the hem of my soul, is joined by the voice that is a friend, softly and steadily narrating a remembrance, a forgotten knowledge of Oneness.

The scale of my world is changing. The texture of Loss rises up a pitted road where I lurch and fall at the forbearance of stones. Once so prominent in the mind, my cultivated identity and achievements now stray from me. Their importance reduces itself each day, while my emerging spirit wanders, inchoate, along a mystic line. In the absence of vanity I fall apart, feel in the tenebrous dark for what I might have known.

Night...

I'm desperate for needed sleep to face tomorrow's treatment. The meter of the clock hands is tireless. It assigns a number to each worry in the dark. Again I invoke the image of Guadalupe.

52

I see myself lying helpless in her arms, the unpremeditated picture of a pietà. As she holds me, I adore her with a conscious, penetrating gaze. With infinite, repetitive grace, her hand moves from her mouth into the cavity of my chest. My tensed body expresses nothing of the finality of death. The apprehension of the image shocks me. Her hand is drenched in my blood. With each slow motion she nurtures herself, feeds on the meat of my heart.

I jerk myself upright. I can't accept this vision of myself. I interpret her actions as abuse, symbolic of my helpless destruction. My mind is running, terrified by the singularity of our union. How can I allow this devouring, feminine appetite for life? Does this ultimate marriage, my arched back and penetrating gaze, her bloody rapture, symbolize the certainty of my early death?

Waking at dawn from a troubled sleep, the attar of the Virgin surrounds me. I long for the succor of her holy and voluptuous embrace, to linger in the folds of her scented arms. Then I remember with fright the claw of her ferocious nature, her long reach, and the red gore of my surrender.

I seek the advice of a Buddhist friend. He tells me the story of a devout monk and his vision. One evening in his old age, as he was meditating on the banks of a river, Kali rose up out of water before him. Slowly filling the sky, she appeared exquisitely beautiful, with red hair flowing the length of her body and her silken robes encrusted with jewels.

The image transfixed him as she spread her legs and began birthing the world. With her hands she pulled forth oceans, mountains, trees, and all the creatures of the planet. Finished creating, she smiled lovingly at the monk. She reached down to earth and scooped up handfuls of newborn babies, one after another, in the thousands.

She brought them to her mouth and ate them with appetite. The monk heard the sound of crunching skulls, the blood running red through the sieve of her teeth. My friend tells me that were it his heart and Guadalupe, he would abandon himself to the moment. He advises me to trust in the heart of the world.

Still...I'm very afraid to open up to something so outside my experience. Different versions of these visual crucifixions keep arriving unannounced. In an effort to ground myself, I have taken to dancing alone as a form of meditation. I'm shocked when the Virgin repeatedly appears in my mind, reaches out and breaks my neck with a single twist of her hand. Is this harsh lesson designed to illustrate the wisdom of regeneration? I'm never harmed or dying. My hypnotic gaze never falters. We are one, together, in this deconstruction and my vulnerability overwhelms me. Demoralized and judgmental, I fall prey to popular psychology. I intellectualize what I fear to feel and define her actions as a violation.

I shutter my imagination and determine to praise less ardent spirits. I banish her, strip the shrine of her artifacts, burn her effigy and dismantle her altar. I do not think of her. I trip and tear a ligament in my ankle on the patio step. Now my world is conveniently safe from soul dancing and its power to open me to her devouring love.

I get a letter from my friend Jim. In it he writes that he believes that we are never born and will never die. I believe that birth and death both involve coming into being. But I don't want to preoccupy myself with this. I need to gain ground in normalcy; too much is slipping away. What I fear most about dying is whether or not I can say goodbye with an open heart. I believe that to occupy a state of grace requires the total release of fear, and I seem incapable of this.

I understand that I inhabit a transformational state influenced by my capacity to surrender to the present moment. I recognize its value, but I want so badly, acutely, to keep living, even without the Virgin's presence near me. Without the influence of her love, I abandon the last mutterings of cynicism. I leave that voice to cry wolf alone, along the faraway edges of my character. My life is up to me.

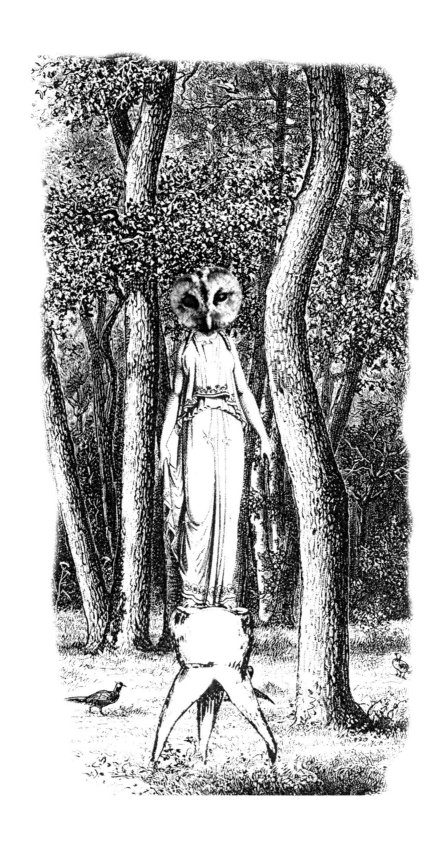

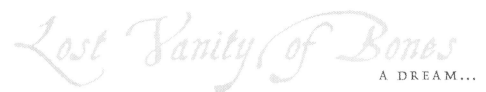

i dream that *I sit alone at the kitchen table eating bread. Swallowing, I notice that a tooth in the back of my mouth is loose. I scout it out with a finger. It falls away at my touch and struggles with my tongue, rolls in forward somersaults toward my lips.*

I spit it out and it lies in full view on my palm, so large in the mouth, so small in the hand. I clamp down on my teeth to test my bite and collapse a bank of molars. I lean over, mouth open, and they fall to the table, a jagged rubble of ivory.

I'm given no respite. I reap my teeth in bitter bundles then suck the lonely sockets of my gums. Hidden wisdoms are all that remain entombed in tissue and bone. I cup my teeth in my hands, a heap of pits, and go in search of others.

I call out in the voice of a desolate woman seen hawking worthless fruit. "Look here! Do you see? I've lost them all. Each tooth, my beauty, my sex! How will I hunt and eat my meat? What have I left to force my will?" I cut my teeth on the root of life, survived by the skin of them. A toothsome woman, fared well in the teeth of it, I bared them in anger and joy. Will I never grow old and long in the tooth nor grind my food with pearls?

I'll plant my teeth in separate graves and water them by weeping. They'll sprout and flourish a pillared forest, white and sturdy as tusks. I'll wander alone this wooded grove, a woman who waits for God, and cut and whittle musical keys to fit in my mouth just so. With these my tongue and fingers play Chansons de Desirenvie, *songs of desire and humble use, attendant to majesty.*

My second chemotherapy treatment is past. Newly bald and feeling vulnerable and ill, I'm fresh from seeking second and third
opinions on stem-cell rescue treatments at various medical centers. In
this process it's taken tremendous energy to command attention as an
individual. Despite this, I'm not at all convinced that I can hope for
personal recognition of my own desires. I'm perceived as a profile and
possible paying customer. Are these doctors capable of factoring personal strengths into my prognosis? Do they understand my
weaknesses? I simply want to talk to them about my life. Their
approval is important.

For my efforts, different medical professionals sum me up in
their pathology reports, in the following ways: "Very pleasant and
informed forty-year-old female patient with stage II, high-risk breast
carcinoma. Although her primary tumor is small (1 cm), there is
involvement of ten axillary lymph nodes, which is the factor that con-
tributes mostly to a higher risk of relapse and death."

"We believe that your prognosis in the absence of treatment
would be for 60–70 percent recurrence within the next five years.
With standard chemotherapy, this would be reduced by approximately
25–30 percent, but with intensive chemotherapy and stem-cell rescue,
there would be a significant improvement in your chances for disease-
free survival. The current data nationwide at three years is an
approximately 75 percent disease-free survival; our own data shows
over 80 percent at two years and 72 percent at three years."

"We feel you are an excellent candidate for this procedure since you are in otherwise good health and are young and vigorous...In addition to the recommendation for intensive chemotherapy, we also would recommend that you have radiation therapy...You were examined by me post-surgery, and I found no evidence of any disease. In addition, you had had multiple studies done including bone scan and CT scan of chest, abdomen, and brain, all of which were negative for any metastatic disease..."

"Thank you for allowing me to take part in the care of this knowledgeable and interesting patient."

My friend takes me to visit her Chinese doctor for a chelation treatment. When we arrive, Dr. Leong is very kindly. He's a small man with rosy cheeks and thinning hair. It is impossible to determine his age. He asks that I write out, on binder paper, my medical history. When he returns, he studies my notes and we discuss my pathology, chemotherapy, stem-cell transplant, genetics and cancer. He is grave. He explains the Chinese medical perspective.

Finally, he sets down all the papers and rests his hands in his lap. He smiles at me and with a penetrating glance he asks, "So, why are you here?" For a moment, I'm speechless. What can he mean; how can he ask that? Isn't it obvious? Or can he see past my pathology to honor my own desires? He can do nothing until I state my own purpose.

What concerns me is my immune system. I would like his help in bolstering it against the chemotherapy. We decide on a chelation treatment and he tests all of the points and meridians in my toes and fingers. Heart, lungs and liver, "Not so bad..." Kidneys, ovaries, immunity, "Very low. Not too good." Dr. Leong looks into my eyes and tells me about his patients. He says, "Spirit go down, immunity go down. Spirit come up, immunity goes up, up. You must be happy, happy, happy, all the time. You take all pills, you do chemotherapy and chelation, you take all supplements, this is the easy part. Spirit, that is the hard part."

As we go to leave, my friend, Dr. Leong and I are alone in the office. My friend says to me, "Becca, did I tell you that Dr. Leong reads palms? Want him to read yours?" I'm curious and elated at the possibility. Dr. Leong's glance at my friend is a withering one. I suppose he feels I may question his professionalism.

Nevertheless, he gently lifts my hand. Each of his gestures is filled with compassion. He looks a long time, turning my hand to gaze at each side. He says, "Ooh, you get over dis cancer, no problem. You see this line? That is your lifeline. It's very long, very straight. You see dis cross, here? Here, somebody broke your life. But you go through that, no problem."

He looks at my friend and points to an upper line in my hand. He says, "Oh, Loma, your friend is so cleva, so intelligent. You see here, she's like you, what is the word, so sentimental, so loyal." He looks at me and says, " Yes. Once you love somebody, you never stop." Once again he studies and exclaims, "You no married! Oohhh." He affectionately slaps my hand in play. "Some lucky guy out dere."

The October Vision

My old friend calls me on the phone. She is someone I have always admired and the mother of two people I cherish. When I was young, I sat at her table. We drank tea and talked with a mutual affection that we still enjoy. I revered this intimacy with her for a second reason. I was in love with her son. I could see his beauty there, in her. She knew my naïve secret and observed me kindly. She is deeply religious. I think back to times when I entered her house on a Sunday morning, scripture blaring from the radio as she made the beds, praying, keeping close to her God. Her faith gives her beauty, radiance and calm. Through it, she judges the world and those around her. She is a rock, a strong woman, and in the steady gaze of her luminous eyes, I have always found a place to be myself. I'm touched to speak with her after so long. She tells me that she learned of my illness from my friend, her daughter, and that she says a prayer for me every day.

It's unlike her to cry, but as she says this, her voice trembles with emotion. She tells me that she is certain I will recover. In her prayers that morning, she witnessed me surrounded by the light of divine presence, so very beautiful and rare. She has seen that I am not alone, instead the center of a devoted hierarchy. I can tell that something big has happened, something very meaningful to her and therefore myself. The emotion she expresses is uncharacteristic of our relationship. I'm very moved by her description of the unexpected vision and the tender and sincere detail with which she has described it. I tell her how much it means to me that *she* sees me in this way.

After our conversation, I remain sitting on the edge of my bed. I don't pretend to know what these experiences mean or if they have a purpose. I just want to stay with my friend's loving, deliberate voice and the depth of hope she has imparted to me, the private gift of her confidence, one woman to another.

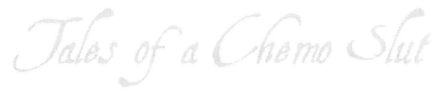
Tales of a Chemo Slut

HISTORIES OF
THE THIRD CHEMO

I spend my days drifting toward the unknown. I give over to heartfelt thinking and revelations portentous as illuminated, shadowy cloud fronts, pregnant with rain. I feel weak and unwell. I can't concentrate. I go from the bed to the couch to the chair. I'm easily moved to tears. I have, all my life, practiced willfulness in the face of God or coherence, however I chose to name it. Now, so humbled, I lose my desire to row toward destiny. I drift and stare up at the sky, keep watches for the burning glimmer of stray angels.

I

Each day is defined by its proximity to a checkup or treatment. Many mornings I travel the hour and back to my oncologist's office. I go for the painful and miraculous shot of Neupren, a drug that raises white cell counts and enhances recovery time after doses of chemo. My right arm is slow to recover sensation and strength. The shortened tendons and constricted veins are maddeningly painful. My macha code finds this frustrating and unacceptable. The high-dose mix of chemo has me looking bad and feeling worse. I look bald and puffy under my hat, feverish without heat. My meat color takes on a gray and pasty hue. My dosage is designed to kill off all the rapidly dividing cells in my body, hair and skin, mouth tissue, and the mucous membrane lining of the intestines and bowel.

In my local grocery store, I'm confused and incredulous before the drug counter's array of intestinal and gastric remedies. I stand in disbelief at the number of options at my disposal. I never realized that Americans were plagued with colossal intestinal turmoil. I join the ranks. Purchasing the packages of hemorrhoid cream and stool softeners, I'm ashamed at the lack of health buying them represents. I'm being given a drug that thins my blood, therefore reducing the chance of infection in my chemo port. I bleed easily and am forbidden aspirin. My dentist has provided me with toothpaste and mouthwash to desensitize my ringing teeth and fragile gums. Fortunately, my earlier torrential nosebleeds have subsided. I begin to lose my eyebrows.

Certain drugs have a universal esthetic effect on the human body: the low slung, hard belly of Thorazine users, the swaying head of heroin, and the swollen moon face of alcoholism. High doses of chemotherapy taint the flesh with toxins and produce what's known as the 'Chemo Look.' With this massacre of cells my body mimics the beauty of the unearthed, of creatures living underground. My translucent face, devoid even of lashes, is bare of pretense, the feminine ego laid waste. I call it my Yeats face, the one given me before the world began. I swear there are days when my ears appear pointed. Yet, I am told that my smile is radiant and suffuses the gray water pallet of my complexion with light.

With the struggle to digest, my once great pleasure of cooking and food diminishes daily. My diet is a mishmash of edible remedies as contradictory as health statistics. Polite, I listen to the testimonies of others' miracle food cures. I try them on, continually reminding

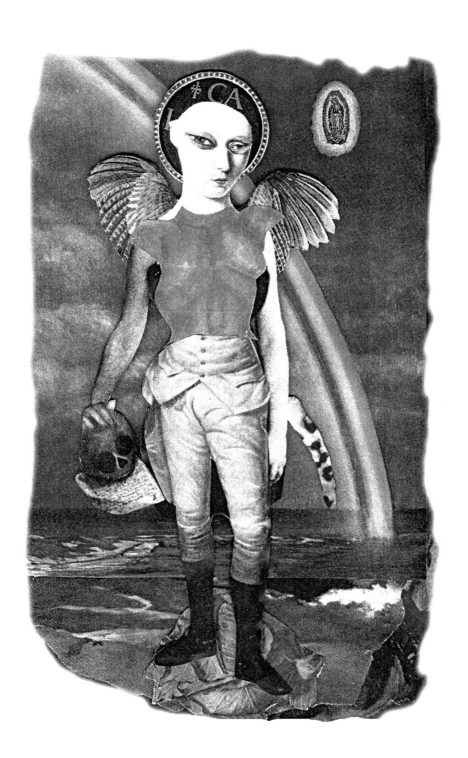

myself that I have low cholesterol and have eaten clean, organic foods for twenty years. I believe diet has little to do with my cancer and therefore radical diet options seem irrelevant. Finally, I settle on eating what's easiest on my liver.

Throughout the day, I swallow combinations of prescription drugs designed to alleviate the side effects of treatments. I combine these with Chinese herbs and medicinal teas. I've lost my appetite for stimulants. The occasional seductions of wine, coffee, cigarettes and joints reside in my memory of carefree, healthy times when I viewed death as optional. I cling to the unaltered preciousness of everyday reality in a body too besieged for drunkenness, or stoned or wired contemplation. I've lost all desire to escape.

Insomnia

again. Midnight and I can't sleep. Paging through magazines in the white light of the bathroom, I listen to my urine echo as it hits the toilet bowl. I'm lonely, but for no one. I roam around the bedroom picking up objects and books. Each one holds a potent memory. I practice detachment and sever my bond with each keepsake and treasured volume with melancholy effortlessness. Material goods have come to hold such little value.

I handle the framed photos on my dresser, pick them up one at a time. I study the faces of people I love and the thought of a solitary, odorless void surrounds me with bone-cracking fear. What will I be without them and why do we suffer the anguish of love and separation? What is life without meaning? I kneel on the floor, tired and filled with the grievous desire to understand. I stroke the graying fur of my sleeping dog and listen to the sonorous music she murmurs, uttering the lost detail of her animal dream.

II

I give in to wakefulness and read by the lamp. At midnight, Edna St. Vincent Millay sonnets; 3 AM Rumi. At four o'clock, I linger over Rilke. Their poems have become my prayers. With the words of the poets to guide me, I've begun to believe in the love expressed by everyone around me. I see its form in every person I encounter with an open heart. My family and friends, the people of my town, hold my hands and look at me with soft, undistracted eyes. Without analysis, I mirror the compassion they give. In these expressions of love and concern, we are one and the same, one body and blood of consciousness. Every day I'm prey to grief and desperation, yet profoundly supported by this love, turned and burnished in its light.

My relationships with loved ones reach an unprecedented resolve. For now, we forgive each other everything. My friends break open my heart with their gestures of selfless concern. I receive marvelous letters and engage in fascinating conversations that connect me deeply with loved ones. The goodness, the fear and often, pretend courage of the people around me, shrivels the twin creatures of cynicism and negativity, replacing them with the green bud of my new life stirring, still in the clutch of its node.

III

Each day I contemplate my impending decision to endure the stem-cell transplant.

I'm rational, then I waver. I research. I reject the treatment and salute it in turns. The insurance company, balking at first, clears an authorization. The doors of my medical journey seem to swing open at each entrance. Every doctor I've interviewed, first, second and third opinion, has recommended me highly as a candidate for stem cell. I read that a large medical insurance company has just paid millions on a lawsuit to a woman denied a transplant. This bodes well for me.

I'm encouraged to undergo the stem-cell treatment as an outpatient and interview with nurses at a cancer clinic. The director is an in-charge sort of woman, who in answering my questions tells me, "You're going to feel like shit, but don't be afraid." I like her forthright manner. But later, after questioning her about the heavy use of antidepressants by ex-transplant patients, I decide I mistrust her. Rather than acknowledge the complexity of the transplant experience, she reacts to my doubts with an aggressive commentary on vitamins and antidepressants being one and the same. No room for nonprotocol here.

Later, awkward as Kafka's scuttling bug, I take my bone-marrow literature in hand. My clanking carapace shields me from the harsh font of the title page. My mouth is dry. I open the book like a lid, repulsed, as though to avoid some dark horror of decomposition. I can barely bring myself to read the explicit details of the stem-cell treatment, every possible adverse reaction described. The details jolt and sicken my senses. The intimate description of side effects stack together in my imagination like dead bodies of a massacre.

A part of me retreats into unawareness. I ask you, how will I do such a thing to myself, cook my blood and encourage the slow, noxious approach of death? To dispel my fears, I get up and yell, sing a loud song for the Gods, "Hey! I'm your transcendental baby." Listen, my friend Al jokes. He calls me a chemo slut. He tells me he's read my number on the wall of a public toilet, "For good chemo, call...."

A Dream of the Father

inside a dream, *I'm running. I see my feet coated with scented, pow-
dery dust. Sagebrush and piñion pine dot the immense landscape. I appear
androgynous in the clothes of a young, old-timey cowboy. Alongside me a
thundering herd of wild horses is also running, the passionate motion of
their dream bodies heroic.*

*I think, how do I manage to keep up with them? I realize that I'm
holding my arm above my head. In my hand is a large Indian smudge, a
smoking incense bundle of sage. I understand then that my running is a
sacred act. I feel at peace and fortified with limitless energy.*

*We run into a town and through the doors of a hospital. Inside, I jog
behind the herd, up a set of stairs. The horses change direction, activating a
chaotic reversal in the stairwell. I leap over the banister to avoid being tram-
pled. In doing so, I realize that I have found what we are there for. I'm here
to witness the euthanasia of "the Father."*

*I step inside his room. His body lies on a stretcher. His chest has been
cut open and his ribs cinched back. He is newly dead. I lovingly lay my
head onto his thighs and look up across the length of his body. With a sense
of joy and curiosity I see that our faces match, except for the incision in my
scalp that is covered by a bandage.*

*I understand as I witness it that the doctors and nurses will remove his
heart and divide it into many pieces. In this way it may be given to the
thousands in need of it. I watch as their bloody hands lift an enormous
heart from his sundered chest.*

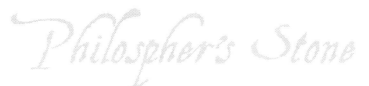
Philospher's Stone

For Justin, Brendan, Gavin, Robert, Mike, John, Jim, Michael, Jaye, Davis,
Charley, James, Chip, Maureen, Kimberly, Julie, Jeani, Amy, Loma,
Gretchen, Jill, Mary and Dinah.

The decision to undergo the stem-cell transplant arrives, unadorned and without fanfare. I have simply run out of time to question my course and the inevitable fruit matures on the vine. The medical insurance coverage, so elusive and faceless, remains a private worry. We are told the transplant is authorized but I receive no written documentation. No papers ever appear bearing the bold headline "Coverage Assured." I can only give my approval of a fate still controlled by anonymous entities.

Several weeks ago, a routine test revealed an antibody for hepatitis C in my system. I firmly believe that I have been exposed and resisted this disease during the last five months of ministrations in hospitals, as it was not detected in the many original blood tests. It puts my recent decision to do the transplant in crisis. So many things could go wrong. I visit my oncologist for a serious and emotional discussion. Because he is a physician who instills trust, I'm able to quell my fears. He doesn't rush my doubts but sits with me for nearly forty minutes. This is an endless time of quiet and reflection to be given by a contemporary doctor whose service is much in demand. I know he believes that, for me, this treatment could be a matter of life or death.

Again, I marry the treatment with the words "I will." I announce my final intentions to suffer the transplant and reflect on the solemn response of loved ones. Outwardly, we appear steadfast, disguising our lack of confidence and anxiety. Inwardly, we brace ourselves for an unfamiliar and frightening reality, spreading like a dark stain on the surface of our imagination.

I visit with post-transplant patients to hear their stories. My conversations with them have been tinged with dread. Feelings of relief, the toxicity of the drugs, the frustration of side effects, the terror of recurrence, the use of antidepressants, are major themes. I'm searching for triumphant stories, joyful responses. I don't find them. Their voices are restrained in their transplant stories, embodying a courageous yet unrequited tone, no treatment warranty upon purchase. Live at your own risk. With me, they are emotionally distant. Like someone who has witnessed an atrocity and wishes to warn of that which defies description. No one mentions fear of an early death directly.

We have little kinship in this fear of pain and dying. Our conversations do nothing to lessen my doubts or bolster my intention. They leave me queasy and ungrounded, as though I have met with phantoms. Instead, our lack of ability to translate the psychological and emotional complexity of our experience elucidates the poverty of our conscripted community. Here, we ring a fire invisible to others, yet sit together as though alone in the darkness. Staring into the dancing firelight, crowded with unspoken questions and desires, we do not address the desperate wonderment we feel in our expectation of a shortened life. The gravity of my decision sits in me with renewed heaviness, shifting its weight like a sleepless nomad.

My perspective of the bone marrow transplant is changing. The transplant treatment is a mythic door of embryonic renewal through which I begin again in the most basic terms. I speak to myself in riddles. I imagine passing through fire and the metaphor of immolation is paramount. I know now that ritualizing the destruction and re-growth of stem cells is the only path that will move me forward.

The dependable metaphor of the phoenix spreads its wings. I think of the terrible drugs as the fiery breast milk of my redemption, a red-hot cauldron of forbidden broth that rewards wisdom for suffering. With my novitiate's hairdo and wasted flesh, I am a disciple of authenticity. I love this life coming to me. I want to arise and go there. Rise up, be the bright-feathered coal shot from ashes, relinquish all wounds, all habits to the past. Through the treatment procedures I'll return to untrained and inspired life.

Can I surrender to any possibility, Death and my desire to live, always with me in the room? I'm beginning to understand that I must rely on my instincts as one would a creed. I understand now that when entering a field of battle, one must set aside all notions. Hesitation breeds fear. Hope can lead to distractions and faith to disappointment. I want to die not in glory, but praising in rapturous gratitude for life.

Repeatedly, I refer to a book of writing by the sixteenth century monk Shosan, sent to me by a friend. In his youth, Shosan had been samurai to the aristocracy. He became a Zen monk at risk of beheading by his lord. He refers to his Za Zen practice as Death Reality, the continuous repetition of the words "I will die," and believes that all creative and spiritual inspiration is best born from a constant meditation on one's own mortality. This rings true to my situation and emboldens me.

Inspired by this thinking, I understand that the triumphant energy I'm seeking resides in the present moment, not in others' stories of the past. I desire to swing my swift sword and free myself from fear, with the idea not that I will beat the cancer but that I will go, exultant, into my own destiny. I want to call Death out and meet it in an open field, knowing that the outcome is either predetermined or beyond my control. Within the lines of this ceremonial dance, life will go on or I will take that mysterious and final journey into intimate knowledge of death and the soul. I find humor in the idea of risking my life to save it and thrill to the opportunity of realizing my ultimate limits.

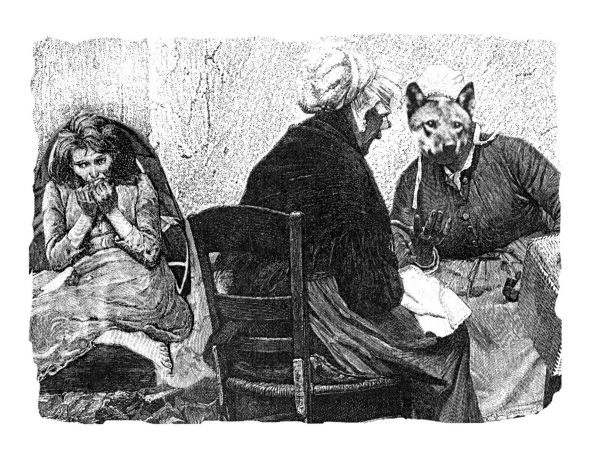

I

The first battle skirmish involves the harvest of my stem cells. These will be gathered from my blood by a transfusion process. I'm told it can take from three to eight days, depending on the health of the patient. The vitality of the stem cells harvested also determines the success or failure of the transplant treatment. I'm nearing the end of my high-dose chemotherapy that began in August. I'm quite weak and I'm having trouble eating.

Today I am certain that I need to create a ritual happening around the stem-cell harvest, a spiritual booster to enliven my cellular activity. I need to raise my chiefs.

For reasons I don't entirely understand, I see these gatherings as two separate events defined by gender, one male and one female. I invite my friends and siblings appropriately with consideration for those I feel would be uncomfortable with this setting. I ask myself, what do I need to learn from the men and women close to me in order to nurture my own courage and vitality? I want to follow their example and be yielding and strong, emotional and decisive, loving and detached. For all of us, it is an opportunity to come together with purpose.

I've decorated the shrine in the garden for Day of the Dead with bouquets of giant cockscomb and marigolds, their resplendent colors a frame for piles of fruit, pictures and candlelight. Mirrored on the surface of the tiny pool is a kaleidoscope reflection of flowers and the smoke of incense. On the crumbling chimney of my patio fireplace, I've painted the triangular stick figure of a neolithic bird goddess of death and regeneration. The ancient caricature I've copied, with bird's feet, cat whiskers and large-set eyes below antennae, is a sovereign presence, part woman, bird of prey and bee.

At twilight, brothers and men friends arrive at my house. Beneath her image, we gather and enjoy a light meal in front of the fire. Myself, my own brothers and men who are brothers to me, form the circle. There are twelve of us. Two more friends, one in Michigan and one in Maine, join us from a distance. The ritual creates a place where they can help me by using their intuition and emotion. The ceremonious playing of saxophones by Gavin and Dave prompts us to the circle by the fire.

What I request from them is mothering. I say that I want to dispel any sense of hopelessness we feel about our inability to protect ourselves and loved ones from illness and death. Then we're silent, humble together, and pray for the ability to embrace what we cannot command. We read from Rilke's *The Book of Hours*. Mike leads us in a meditation. Although we don't speak of it directly, each of us attempts to renew our faith in an inherent goodness in the universe. Just being together and silent brings us so close. We visualize my vibrantly healthy stem cells and meditate for twenty minutes.

At the ringing of bells, we stretch and talk, eyes bright by the light of the fire. Mike says to me, "I kept seeing you, the way you deal with the cancer, like a creature hunting or trotting through woods and grass, alert, nose to the ground." We laugh, and then everyone is quiet for a time. Suddenly, we hear a fox barking from the woods above the patio and we break into amazed laughter at such an auspicious greeting. We sing together in harmony, talk to each other. We tell stories and drink tea. We end with another simple ritual. Each of us throws into the fire a symbolic object representing what we no longer wish to carry. We joke and laugh some more, then say good night. The strength and tenderness of these men, our love for each other, lifts me up, and I feel alive and protected. My head on the pillow, I close my eyes and rest, beyond the grasp of fear.

II

The next day, my friend Maureen invites women friends of mine to her home. First, we have lunch. All of us present love to eat, one sign of our astonishing vitality. As we sit around the table, I feel a bit removed and sadly reserved amongst so much beauty. My colors are muted and my spirit more tolerant than celebratory. I'm fatigued after last night's gathering and am aware of holding my energy together. I feel too ill to eat my food, but I take enormous pleasure in watching these women I love so deeply feast and talk with one other. We tell stories from the past and review the history of our friendships.

Dishes done, we walk together through the woods to a large meadow. The autumnal grass and trees are sunlit in thickened layers of Van Gogh yellow. We wander silently, captivated by the dry scent of Indian summer air. Crows caw from a stately oak at the grass line, discussing us and formalizing our mood. We sit on blankets in a circle. My friend Loma leads us in a meditation.

It catches me off guard when I'm asked to lie in the middle of the circle. I'm afraid to feel too much. Yet I want all of us to give up our striving toward power and identity, our need to be recognized. I want simply to be together for these transient moments, turn softly like leaves to sun, toward our intuition and receptive spirit.

There is no need to ask or even wish. As I lie here, my friends lay their hands on me while Loma speaks to them in a hushed voice.

Then all of us are quiet for a time. The crows settle themselves on branches. In the silence of the meadow and a breeze that rustles the dry grass, my friends' emotions surface. Their tears fall on each other's hands. I lie here in the October sun, my frail body held by women I love. My eyes are closed and my heart is overflowing. The muffled sound of their tears, the responsiveness of their touch, thaws a place in myself I have never known. I allow them to reach me and I lie in the womb of us. I behold the quality of love being given me. These women are rare people of dignity and passion. They call on their own courage and feed me with its power.

Afterward, we read poetry and talk until we depart the meadow in unbroken silence. Amy and Jeani, their arms linked in mine, help me to walk up the hill, back to the house. There, amidst much bawdy laughter, we sit together again and quickly consume a large frosted cake.

Now, more than any other time, I feel I am living my life within the divine body of love. I bow untroubled before my family and my friends. I gain a certain peace toward the world's suffering. I realize that I've spent my life avoiding what I perceived as the pain and terror of capture in the net of attachment. Now I rest with weight against its fiber and understand the truth of love again. This awakening in gratitude frees me from the wasting corruption of fear. The rituals have roused me to wonder and I return to myself filled with innocence and courage. With this love in my heart, I discover what I desire. I seek to find serenity in battle.

Blood Harvest

I am not Valkyrie or Amazon, Medusa or Dragon, Crusader or Penitent. My passions are temperate. Still, I recognize my opportunity of cancer to grasp the heroic quest. I am Wounded and Nurse, Captor and Slave in a chronicle of my own making. What news can be birthed into a ravaged world without a mytho-poetic journey of the self?

These are the ideas I dwell on at the stem-cell harvest, once again entwined with technology as with a lover. One of the classic metaphors of the Hero's journey is a harvest of blood. The willingness to blood-let in battle, to give of the liquid of life, makes possible the eventuality of a healed wound. Will this process confirm my faith in continuum? A stem-cell harvest is, in effect, a major blood transfusion. It is a pain-less procedure, except for the insertion of a tube into my subclavien vein. I've been told this will be "uncomfortable," doctor-speak for "it will hurt like a son of a bitch."

Ironically, it's Halloween. The nurses move about energetically cracking jokes and prepping me for the insertion surgery. One of them wears a pink plastic mold of female buttocks on the backside of her uniform. Humor runs high on the ward as other nurses and interns come by to view her costume. I'm in a high-strung state of mind and influenced by this. The room suggests a stage full of actors, a troupe of chatty mummers defrocked of satin and bells. In my mind, the medical procedure is transforming itself. I see it as a highly ritual-ized act. For no other reason but to make it juicy and rich, I invite the impulses of my imagination to distill themselves into meaning. I value the metaphors. I can't believe how weird and symbolic it seems that the date of my blood transfusion and cell harvest would fall on All Hallows' Eve.

The surgeon arrives to place the port and tube into my chest. The nurses politely escort my mother out of the room. The young man lying next me, in his eighth day of harvesting, disappears behind the swift clatter of the bed curtain pulled by the nurse. The surgeon introduces himself as I lie on my back looking up at him. He tells me that what he is about to do will be painful. I must be fully alert during the procedure in the event that my lung is nicked or punctured by the deep insertion of the tube.

He hesitates and inspects the width of the one provided. He objects, saying it's too large a size for the small frame of my upper body. He goes in search of one that is more correct, but returns empty-handed and reaches for the original. The nurses brace my forearms and ankles as the surgeon cuts a slice in the anesthetized skin on my chest.

At the first pressure of insertion, he raises his voice and loudly commands my attention. As it penetrates my chest, the tube size begs comparison to a shovel handle through the heart of a hummingbird, the force of it startling up the metaphor of rape.

I hear myself whimper and
cry out with the overwhelming inclusion of the tube.
In a numbing impulse, my whole body seizes upwards toward my chest. The
thunderous voice and the pressure of hands keep me from disassociating. The booming
voice asks, "Are you a Democrat or a Republican? What, I can't hear you? Are you mar-
ried? You're tough, you're really tough, are you a mother? You must be a mother. No? It's
easier if you've been in labor. I thought you'd been in labor. Where are you? Come back.
Are you with me?" I think, do torturers use this shouting technique, how can he do this
job, day in and out? I approach the question, when do you beg for mercy? I feel drug
about, mauled and speared by the tooth of a great beast.

The surgeon tells me, "Good job," and pats my leg. The nurse cleans up my blood and attends me. Another dries my tears. My body lies rigid and galvanized by the trauma. A shunt juts from my chest, waving a tentacle of tubes. A nurse administers a shot of morphine and the effect is immediate. I feel my hands unfurl their grip. The procedure has lasted all of ten or twelve minutes. Propped up by morphine, tense and drawn from pain, I will be occupied with the harvest for six or seven hours more.

An awkward sense of intimacy crops up between the young man in the next bed over and me. I imagine how he must have cringed, overhearing the struggle. Underneath our sparse conversation lies the deep familiarity of strangers in a shared drama. The surgeon's analogy was right: it is as though this man witnessed my labor pain in the birthing of these cells to light. We talk a little bit, but the morphine makes conversation difficult. I return to my effort of concentration on the transfusion process. The success of the upcoming transplant lies

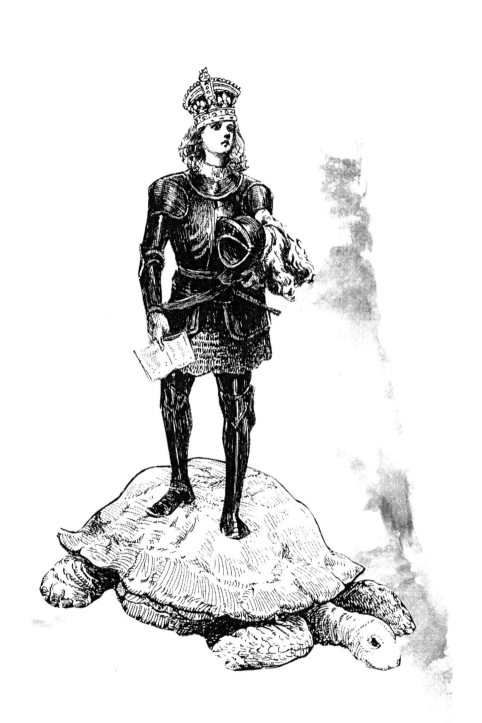

in the potency and health of these fleeing cells. I pray for the courage to believe in them.

When it's time to go, I slide from the bed and reach for my sweater and the morphine hits me in a wave of nausea. I vomit in the sink near the hospital bed. I vomit in the parking lot and the hotel toilet. I vomit through the night, each contraction of my chest prompting a misery of surgical pain. The next morning, I'm so weak I find it difficult to walk. Having nursed me through the night, my mother tenderly helps me to the car. As I arrive for my second day of harvesting the hospital staff hooks me to a replenishing IV. As they work, they give us the good report. In one day, not the expected three to five, they've harvested all the stem cells necessary for the transplant. To their delight and astonishment, I've gushed forth a fountain of healthy newborns.

I feel sure that we've influenced this collection of cells with our meditations, our faithfulness and the acceptance of circumstances beyond our control. My imagining soul lifts and rises in praise of the news. Oh you, my seeds of tender shoots, soon to be nurtured by ashes, I give you up into the mystic heart of being, sheathe the sword of my imagining and pass weak and triumphant from the grisly field.

At the Grave of Love

zooming into my *dream from a distance I see two figures standing together talking. I recognize myself, and my once beloved, in the midst of a Gothic graveyard. We stand in the shadow of a church wall whose damp mortar breathes a halo of moisture around us. At our feet are two freshly dug mounds of earth. The black silhouettes of enormous trees tower above. Their branches bend to embrace us, scraping and listening. The night sky is a bruise of shifting clouds lit up by a brilliant moon. Its bluish radiance reflects an eerie glow on tombs and statuary. Nearby, a white robed angel, brandishing a sword, blinds us with her marble light.*

I'm dressed in the mourning clothes of a Greek widow. My face, illuminated as the angels, is framed by the fringe of a turbaned headscarf, black as the dress, shawl and shoes that camouflage my body in the darkness. My bald face, and my hands floating before me, appear autonomous in the black night.

The beloved is naked, but his long blond hair hangs like a shimmering cowl about his head. He engages me in a deeply intimate discussion. We bend our shoulders toward each other in conspiratorial concentration. He steps back, faces me with authority. He dictates, "You do it like this. Watch me." He lies down on the surface of one of the mounds and I feel a disquieting pathos at the sight of his thin white body.

He begins to vibrate his limbs in the fine soil of the grave. An expression of horror distorts my face as his features and hands transform themselves into those of a Nosferatu. His teeth are long and his fingers clawlike. As he quivers, the soil climbs his skin with a terrible velocity. In moments, it covers all but a few locks of shining hair that lie displaced, a misbegotten constellation whose light no longer has the capacity to guide.

Love lost, a panic rises in me, opens my mouth and forms a mute black hole of screaming. Then the winged creature arrives. Spiraling down from the sky above me, his batlike form has the face of a stone gargoyle. His hairy dragon wings are small and well formed. His appendages resemble those of a crustacean with large pitted pinchers for hands.

With him comes deafening music that overwhelms the landscape, absorbing everything osmotically. I stand consumed by this choir of thousands, this opera of the psyche that honors and grieves the end of love. The harmonic voices arrive from the root of ancient times in a layered, dissonant chanting of the syllabic ahh, *the notes traveling backward summoned from their capture in the speed of light.*

The creature swoops low and lifts me by the back of my dress. My benign Hermes, no menace in his heart, carries me with a delicate and purposeful grip. I hang from underneath his body like a broken doll, arms dangling. My head hangs to one side and my eyes are blank. My mouth still shapes the hole but through it comes my voice, a throaty moan that joins in the singing. Every cell of my body is permeated with the song that stabs and lifts me on its blade, my body possessed by sound.

We fly in slow silhouette against the light of dawn, through the open doorway of my house and into the darkened kitchen. The creature holds me in the air near the ceiling until I realize that we are not alone. My sleeping brother wakes and leaps from the couch, turns on all the lights and

87

demands to know who is there. The creature drops me to the floor, delivered, beats his wings and is gone. My brother finds me crouched behind a table leg. I wink up at him, deceive him with a smile and shrug. I keep the knowledge of my encounter to myself. It's best to fake normalcy and go on.

IV. MARROW IN THE BONE

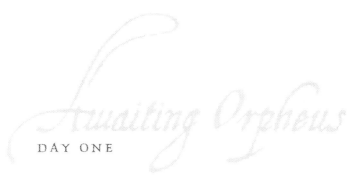

Awaiting Orpheus

DAY ONE

I enter the isolation room for the first time through a darkened vestibule where elaborate hand-washing rituals are performed. There, gowns, masks, gloves and other isolation-room paraphernalia are grouped in dimly lit clusters appropriate to their use. The few nurses and visitors who will enter and exit stop here for a last cleansing. A round window in the heavy door at one end will allow me a glimpse of those too germ-exposed to enter. As I push open this door and penetrate my sunlit room, I recall the comment of a woman I spoke with who had gone through a transplant: "It was like being shot into space...unknown territory." I think of the room then as my new planet and explore it as such, step by step. Within a day or two there will be no stopping what I have put in motion, no easy exit of my own accord.

Unpacking pajamas and socks, I grasp the magnitude of what has occurred in this room over time. I sense an aura of physical pain made memorable by the sympathetic gestures of others, a stage set where one drama after another is enacted. Here, there will be no birdsong or comfort of light and leaves. This starched and sterile bed will be mine to suffer in and accept the care and kindness of strangers.

I sit down and allow my eyes to drift along the parameters of the room and begin to understand how pronounced the obvious, inherent loneliness of illness may become. I realize, in the midst of abundant, loving support, a part of me will privately remain an animal, shedding its skin in a secluded corner.

Nurses busy themselves in a new and painful insertion of a second chemo port on the opposite side of my chest. Tentacles of small tubes harness me to a rolling metal IV stand, my dance partner for the next eighteen days. From the hanging bags come one line for nourishment, one for poison, another for pain. There will be no feed lines of joy or spirit. The medicine of sacred interaction must come from the heart of all of us, strangers and kin, whose compassion will sustain our beliefs and make many things possible.

My sister busies herself all day seeing to my comfort. My niece and nephew have made a paper Christmas tree that she tacks to the wall in a hopeful effort of cheeriness. Christmas cards and posters of paintings by Van Gogh brighten empty walls. I fill the drawer by my bed with photos of loved ones to be near at hand when the hours are longest. Maggy leaves late and reluctantly, knowing her loving concern and courage are the only gravity on this unknown planet. Alone, in the hospital dark, I feel doll-sized, dwarfed by circumstance and the surrender of my will, afraid and in pain in a strange bed.

I tell myself I'm here because I was able to convince myself to do the unthinkable. I did this by making metaphor and meaning of an undesired reality. My ability to endure is in direct correlation to my faith in divine presence. Success is not a matter of outcome. The only measure of success is my capacity to accept what is given minute by minute. I close my eyes in a futile imitation of sleep. Over the humming quiet of medical equipment, my imagination hears Mahalia

Jackson, singing swinging gospel to the unformed fears in the back of my brain, "Keep your hand on the plow, oh Lord."

In the morning, nurses arrive and explain the protocol again. I'll be given maximum doses of chemotherapy drugs for four days in a row and over the weekend the side effects of the drugs will emerge. At the start of the second week, my original stem cells will be returned to my bloodstream. I'll wait an undetermined amount of time, approximately eight to fifteen days, for my stem cells to rediscover my bone marrow, engraft themselves there and begin to reproduce. Stem cells are invisible to the naked eye. It is not known how they return to the bone marrow. On faith alone I must embrace their mysterious motivation.

The stew of drugs they give me is astonishing. The chemotherapy itself is a combination of three drugs whose side effects can include: skin irritation, swelling, complete loss of hair and nails, mouth sores, radical sore throat, vomiting, mood fluctuations, slurred speech, changes in vision, dissolving of the mucous membrane lining, difficulty in breathing and bladder irritation. Major disruption of hormone production resulting in sterility is certain. Damage to the heart and the development of leukemia and other cancers are also possible.

Combined with the chemo, I'm given anti-nausea drugs, including Ativan as a tranquilizer and sleep medication, painkillers and several broad-based antibiotics. I'm also given a powerful drug that represses herpes zoster, known as shingles. Another drug is administered to protect the lining of my bladder. I'll use medications to reduce mouth sores and Lidecane as a gargle for the pain of rawness in my mouth and throat.

The nurses insist that I shower once or twice each day with super-strength antibacterial soap to cleanse my skin of the residual drugs being released through my pores. What troubles me most is the prospect of taking morphine, the centerpiece drug of the doctor's protocol. The intense vomiting I experienced, induced by morphine during the stem-cell harvest, is not something I wish to repeat. I've requested an alternate drug. The nurses tell me that my request has been denied but that the doctor has approved a slightly lower dose, to which they will add Benadryl to up the potency of the pain-killing mix.

I'm unable to sleep. With my eyes closed, I can still perceive the small red, green and yellow lights of the beeping monitors that surround my bed. On top of the morphine and other drugs, I've been given two strong tablets of Benadryl. I'm very high, unpleasantly intoxicated. As sleep evades me, my anxiety mounts. I want to thrash and turn, but the shunt of tubes in my chest makes this painfully impossible. My body responds to the sensation of drifting toward sleep as spiraling in a vortex down, down, downward, then jerking awake as though terrified of drowning. Something is crawling up the pole of the IV stand. The ceiling is crawling, undulating with large, hard-backed insects. I feel them hit my legs when they drop, in squadrons, onto my bed...

Upset by my night of hallucinogenic interludes, I've requested to see the doctor.

Instead, the head nurse pays me a visit. I tell her that my sensitivity to drugs makes it difficult for me to tolerate the pain-medication protocol. I cannot go through another night like last night. I attempt to explain how important it is for me to remain in touch with myself. I want to know what is happening to me, not only externally but internally as well. The nurse explains with a kind of forced patience that most people in my situation prefer not to know what is happening to them. She cannot protect me from the experience I'm to go through without the morphine.

Exasperated, she warns me that she can't be responsible for my pain and discomfort if I refuse to submit to the protocol. What if I suddenly lapse into severe pain? It might be hours, days, before medication I request could be approved, be administered and effectively satisfy potential conditions I might face.

I explain that it is a risk I want to take. We finally compromise with the decision to allow the smallest dose of morphine possible to administer but one I can't really detect. In turn, I must agree to a level strong enough to protect the hospital from accusations of neglect should I fall prey to my own desires.

I have already discussed an alternative to doping with the two main nurses in charge of my care. They advise me that within several days, I will be unable to swallow even liquid. When this happens, they will rig me with a suction device of the type used by dentists that will remove the saliva from my mouth, saving me the discomfort of swallowing. This device, combined with the anesthetic Lidecane gargle, should keep me relatively comfortable. It is their view that if I handle the treatment well, avoiding high fevers, severe throat sores or other complications, I should be able to do without high doses of pain medication. If I begin to show signs of struggle, they will be the first to recommend more drugs.

A nurse is attempting to flush the tube to my chemotherapy port. Her hand slips.

The tube dislodges itself, wakes and writhes around, spitting poisonous liquid near my face. It sprays sea-blue-colored drugs on her uniform and my sheets. She jumps back and presses the red emergency button by the side of my bed. In split seconds, other nurses appear. They rush in and immediately help me from the bed, strip my blankets, sheets, and gown, then assist the nurse in rapidly removing the top of her pantsuit uniform. Comfortably back between clean sheets, I ponder this priority drill. I cannot allow myself to dwell on the now obvious toxicity of the drugs coursing through my veins.

For the last several nights, I've been working on a collage with papers and scissors I brought with me to the hospital. Collage is my art medium of choice and the images I create are full of symbols and metaphors. Tonight I finish an image I know will be difficult for me to look at in the future. In a black and white photo, an outstretched hand rests amongst sand and stones. Along the surface of each finger and ending at the nail run fluid lines of red, the texture of which appears to vibrate, resembling crowds of blood-filled cells. On the back of the hand lies a newborn child in a golden, egg-shaped globe.

Surrounding the globe are pale blue tears that form a fringe for the hand where it lies. The image reflects my mind full of struggle, suffering and rebirth.

The drugs are beginning to blur my vision so that reading is difficult. The scissors have also become awkward and heavy in my weakened hands. Despite this, the collage work is so sustaining that I begin another, this one for my oncologist back home. On the tape deck I play the soulful voices of Nina and Mahalia, Betty, Billie and Etta singing, keeping me in the blue mood of the heart. My sister and mother arrange a schedule and family and friends faithfully come and go, bringing fresh and loving energy to me.

This treatment has become a vocation, the work I do with the help of others, especially my sister. Being confined to my hospital room has ceased to trouble me. The bathroom is as foreign a country as I care to go. I avoid the picture window. For me, the gray city street below belongs to a world out of time. I want to stay with the feelings inside me, the love that seems to saturate the aura of this room. The lonelier my moments and the more acute my physical discomfort and emotional anxiety become, so deepens my connection to this stillness, this sense of compassionate rapture that pervades my being.

Distracted as I am with these sensations, I fail to warm to the physical therapist assigned to my case. He arrives for visits with a stretchy rubber exercise tool, which I am instructed to use while lying in bed. I feel repulsed by the thing and its colorful affiliation with a future vanity.

The therapist carries a checklist and wags his finger at my lack of interest. I know that his program is altogether reasonable, but cannot move myself to participate in such a radical shift in mentality. He is the only person with whom I feel distressed. How can I explain that it is not necessary for me to save myself from decline, that I lie curled in the arms of divine love and do not wish to shift my position, that my life in the future holds no fixed importance? How can I show him that should he stop and listen, lay his burden down and curl up beside me, we, like Beethoven, might hear music in silence?

My oldest brother arrives at six. His handsome, smiling face is rosy with the cold. He delicately lifts my hand and holds it between his calloused, work-worn fingers. He is a person who loves nature and chooses to live a rustic life. His face filled with radiant sweetness, he kisses me on my hairless head. His hair is still short. He had it buzz-cut when I lost mine, in an act of solidarity. He tells me excitedly about the reflections of Christmas lights in the rain puddles outside. He describes what he ate for dinner and shows me the art magazines he's brought me. He announces that our seed catalogs have arrived in the mail as he settles into the chair by my bed. He is a guide who rides with me into mystery, the priest and philosopher traveling with me on this quest. During the months of my illness, after digesting the implications of my diagnosis, we've discussed Buddhism, death and meditation, cancer theory and mysticism.

Tonight he appears calm and full of ready energy, curious about me. I ask him to read aloud. My friend has sent some of his newly published poems. I want to generate some feelings, eat his words with my ears: luxurious, imaginative swallowing in a throat too swollen for food.

Justin is masterful at reading poetry. When I was in junior high, he brought home the writings of Gary Snyder, Lew Welch, Robert Bly, Sylvia Plath, Charles Olsen, Kenneth Patchen, Anne Sexton, Richard Brautigan, Emily Dickinson and Kenneth Rexroth. During a time of salmon fishing work in Arcata, he sent me xeroxed copies of Charles

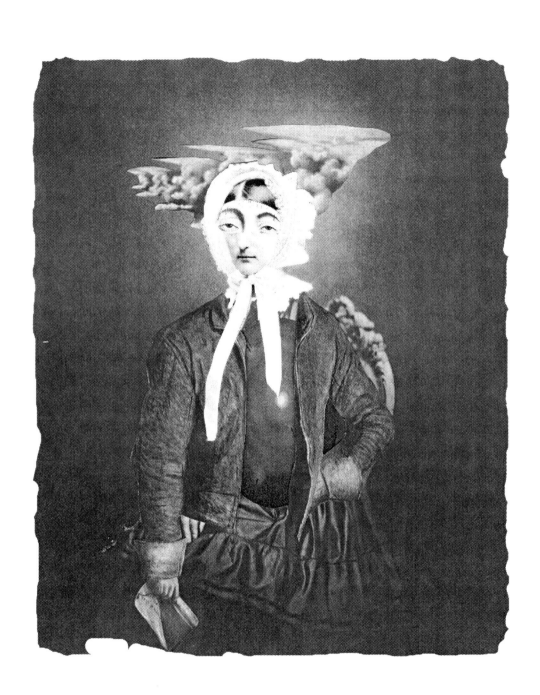

Simic poems. Now, hunched in the big chair, he ruminates, mutters expressively over various sequences. Then, finalizing his selection, he clears his voice and with force begins to read these Harrison poems.

He learns each one. Reads them aloud, two or even three times in a row. Each rendition of the poem he reads offers a new perspective, a different rhythm or subtle inflection. Periodically, he lifts his free hand, waves it as though conducting. He looks at me, his face bright and grinning with wit. He shakes his head in awe at the beauty of the words. After a particularly grand passage concerning the numerous spines of an Ocotillo cactus framing a desert dawn, he looks over at me humorously and says, half jokingly, half seriously, "I don't know, Bec. The energy in the room is, you know," he laughs and rolls his eyes, "filling up, wouldn't you say? Dare we continue?"

Suddenly, not ten seconds later, there is a loud, wrenching crash from the street outside. After it comes the sound of a shower of glass hitting the pavement. Justin leaps from the chair to the window to describe the scene below, a dramatic fender-bender with no apparent injuries. We look at each other and burst out laughing.

Alone, late into the night, the room is at peace with me. The spirits here have listened in on my brother's eloquent voice reading the truth of poets. They, with us, honored beauty. Together in this place we shared a transient perception of the world. We are all of us but the seeds of meteorites planted in the dust of stars.

Blossoms from Fire

I

    After four brutal doses of chemotherapy, my bone marrow has been dying over the weekend. I'm left with little immunity and the side effects of the drugs erode my calm and comfort. Two special technicians arrive to transfuse my stem cells back into my bloodstream. Stem cells of mine collected in October have been mixed with my own plasma and further combined with a freezing solution and DMSO as a preservative. The two women set up a small station next to my bed. Quickly, they thaw each frozen bag of stem cells and hang them one at a time from my IV stand. The contents are fed through the catheter in my chest, along with other drugs to help with nausea and side effects. The smell of the DMSO is overpowering. Like skunk spray in a closest, the odor infects everything in the room. The fluid is freezing cold in my veins and the accompanying nausea manifests itself as a gag reflex I can barely control. I feel swept up in the force of the experience, woven to a loop-de-loop at the county fair. The process takes several hours. By the time it's completed I'm exhausted and cannot lift my head from the pillow or relate to others. My mother and brother have arrived and sit by me while I fade in and out for the rest of the day.

By now it's obvious to me that, at best, my nights will be filled with fitful catnaps. Nurses check my vital signs every hour or so, registering my weight and temperature and measuring my limbs for swelling. These nightly activities, combined with a day of lethargy, make achieving REM sleep next to impossible. The significant dreams I've hoped for are lost to me. My brother-in-law, John, brings me a CD of French medieval songs of courtly love and wonderment sung by Anne Azema. Listening to her ethereal voice singing each song over and over and over through the hours is how I navigate my sleepless nights. The vaulted, echoing quality of her voice, with its essence of medieval mysticism, is music that best describes the state of my soul. No other music I know could transport me, hold me like this, in the way I wish to be held.

I am in love's embrace. Lying in bed drifting in and out of thought, or waking to find my sister, one of my brothers or my mother sitting by my bed, sustains me. The love and concern in the faces of a few dear friends allowed to visit is food on which I stay strong. This afternoon, waking from the spent blossom of sleep, I opened my eyes to see my parents in chairs at the end of my bed, silently looking into each other's faces. I will remember this forever. How can I describe the depth of courage summoned, not by me but by my community, for hope of renewal and grace?

II

My mother brings me a package. I open it to find a beautiful cer-
tificate that represents a donation made in my name to Expedition
Inspiration. The women members of the expedition are all cancer sur-
vivors. They intend to climb the highest mountain in the western
hemisphere. A Tibetan prayer flag with my name inscribed will travel
with them to the summit. Women friends, coworkers from my job,
have made the donation. After reading the enclosed booklet, I realize
that the expedition has already arrived at the mountain base camp.
The thoughtfulness of my friends fills my eyes with tears. I think of
my flag on the summit, loosening prayers with every rustle and whip
of mountain wind, the perfect gift of inspiration.

III

Nearly every morning, I awake to the sound of the young man in the room next to mine, the same man who was next to me during my stem-cell harvest. I listen to the violence of his vomiting. His suffering seems horrible to me and the long silences between periods of retching is unbroken by talk or laughter. He has very few visitors. I question the nurses about his condition. This morning I call him on my phone to talk and sympathize, but the discrepancy between our conditions becomes embarrassing to me. It's clear that he is much more ill than I. He's nearing the end of his treatment and sounds desperate and angry that his doctors are refusing to release him on the date he expected. In my condition, his trouble is more than I can assimilate. I don't call again, but hold him in my thoughts and send the spirit of kindness like a ghost through the wall.

A fellow woman patient recovered enough from her transplant to walk the hall outside my room waves through the round window in my door in poignant encouragement. I love her for this, yet it distresses me. I don't have the energy or desire to project myself into the future. I am living moment to moment. I don't want to think of the struggle to recover that lies ahead.

IV

I am without acute pain. My throat is closed, so drinking is very difficult. I have not had solid food for five days. My mouth is a woolen chamber, a fuzzy sponge, where my teeth leak tiny rivulets of blood. It is a place deserted by pleasure. My lack of sleep is devastating. The skin is numb on my back and arms where my pores are still sweaty with poison. I associate this absence of sensation in my skin with death. The itchiness of my numbed skin riddles me with anxiety and intense discomfort. But all of this is not too bad. It's the weakness I feel that frightens me. How close will I come to the lifeless grave? I lie adrift, my moorings lost, a branch of yellow leaves that the touch of a fingertip makes fall.

My friend Julie delivers this postcard to the hospital: "You are in my heart. I woke up last night feeling a very strong connection to you, then fell back to sleep and dreamed that I went to the hospital and took your place for the afternoon to serve some of your time there. This morning I listened to the Campanile chime eight for the Becca meditation. Mike and the girls still have colds...We send you much love, couragio."

One day drifts into another in a hazy zone between sleep and wakefulness. Members of my family are in attendance through all hours of the day. In one difficult moment, I learn by phone that a friend, diagnosed with breast cancer just before I entered the hospital, has had a mastectomy.

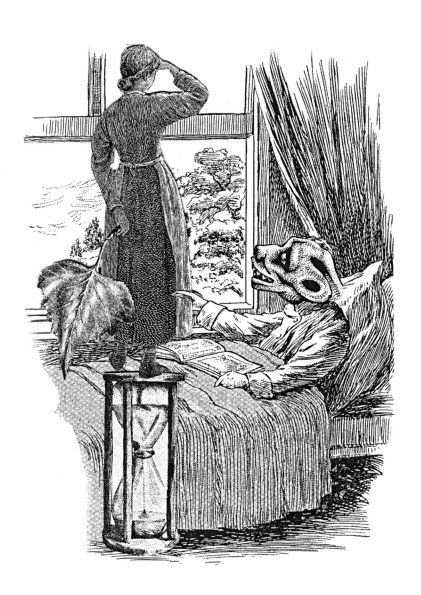

DAWN
DECEMBER 18, 1994

I open my eyes to see the first rays of dawn light

along the hem of the curtain. At the same moment, I sense the pal-

pable presence of Death sitting in the chair next to my bed, just the two of

us, sensing and waiting.

My visitor is a male persona, a sound and an abstract darkness. He is filtered

light embodied in discordant vibration kindred to the buzz of insect wings. This high-

pitched tone, full of formless energy, interacts with the molecules dying in and around

me.

A sudden tidal breath of mist covers my face. Now a sea grotto filled with lapping

waves, he is cool and freshened darkness penetrated by pinholes of brilliant, terrify-

ing light. Blinded by sensation, I blink and cover my eyes. There is nothing I can

do except recognize the futility of escape. As though the visitor had a face

and eyes, we nod, bow together in the acknowledgement of my

incontestable mortality. Then the presence is gone, Leaving

behind a bit of atomized air in his place.

DECEMBER 19, 1994

Members of my family have traveled to attend the wedding of my youngest brother. My friend Kimberly comes to watch over me. I spend the day with her in a series of cathartic episodes of emotion, euphoria and grief in between periods of drifting sleep.

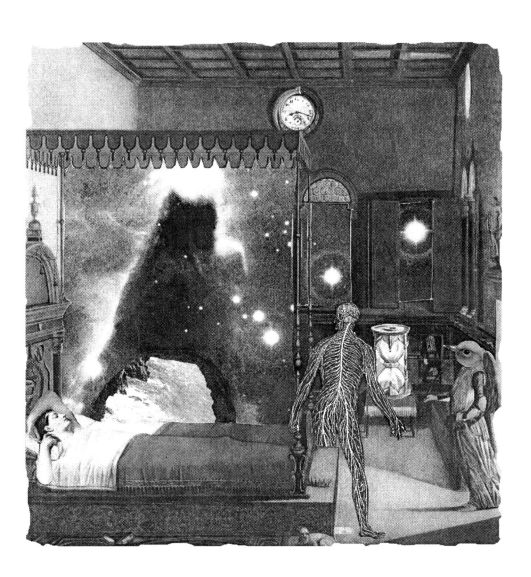

Every simple remembrance between us, the Rilke she reads me, my dear friend Mike, who waves from the window in the door, sets me to open weeping. Kimberly ignores the nurses and lies down on the bed and holds me. We cry and then laugh together. We wag our heads and chortle some more at the impossible nature of life, how the desire to understand gets in the way of awareness.

My beautiful, redheaded friend knows the value of strong emotions. With her I can open to my truest self, as we both understand vulnerability as a creative act. I know that my behavior alarms and upsets her but that she won't interfere or discourage me. My illness has been a table laden with a feast of misfortune. We have eaten of it and digested it together with cameras and canvases. She has taken my portrait as I am, bald, with a pearl choker and droplets, in a red velvet evening gown, low cut, where my chemo port protrudes undisguised. Don't be repulsed, because she found me beautiful and captured that in her lens. In the photograph I appear blooming, proud and undiminished. She has taken my picture many times, in many guises, over the years. Because she believes in me, this portrait will become just one more of many that artfully document our lives on paper. When we cry together, we always laugh.

From where has this weeping come? Is it grief for the last vestige of my youth, the end of an era, or more? Could it be the rainy spring sky of my new life that washes clean the grimy face of all regret? The nurse's chart notes for this day read, "In good spirits."

The Vigor of the Graft

For Gavin, Maria and Julian

I

Asleep an hour, I wake abruptly at 4 AM. For several days now, an unfamiliar scent has hung in the air around my bed, a tincture of chemicals and flesh. My skin is imbued with the subtle colors of an aging bruise, smudgy hues of gray, yellow and sea green. My swollen limbs lie weighty against the sheets, sunken, like sodden mushrooms in fallen leaves, newly rotting after a heavy rain.

Despite my severely enervated state, I wake restless and wide-eyed. I tilt my face as though to sniff the air. Struggling up, I shuffle into the bathroom with its wretched, glaring light. Mouth care. I untangle myself from the IV stand and gargle with the Lidecane, letting the sink hold my weight as I spit. The mirror in the bathroom is unforgiving; rather than glass, its surface is highly polished stainless steel. More alien in appearance each day, I'm science made manifest. My puffy face is at the same time strangely sunken. My nose and chin reach for one another between my swollen, poison-bloated cheeks. My ears are alarmingly pointy. In the sulpha-colored tile bathroom, the reflection of my bald face is the color of cheap French mustard. I gaze at my reflection with slightly forced compassion, sardonic. "Sweet Mother, can't go no further down than this and live."

Yet...some obscure energy has arrived in me. I make my way back to the bed, collapse there from exertion, eyes open. I listen to the pounding of my quickened heart. I see a vision of myself striding, unstoppable, across a high, windy, limitless plain. My form is gigantic, naked. A towering muscular body of polished petrified wood, striped, the grain marks visible as dark veins. My mane of hair blows about. My slow and ponderous feet shake the ground. (SHE is coming).

II

Then, moonlight washes a shadow landscape of falling leaves, bare trees, the dark bodies of conifers and the mulched and leaf-littered ground. Naked, I crouch there, alert in the tinselly light. A thin band of mottled fur runs along my spine; my long tail probes and stiffens. I have been hunting in the silver night. I have been running on all fours.

I deafen myself with endless panting, hu, hu, hu, hu, Hu, Hu. Soft at first, building to a deafening volume, until...fleet! Fleet! My being is flooded with the freedom of boundless energy. I'm running again, blurred jumping, fierce whipping through branches. My lungs and heart pound in a passionate, metered embrace. I need no destination, no supply, all thought maternal. My instincts have been born of fire. (SHE is with me!)

III

The night nurse greets me at dawn. "How you doin', honey? I got good news. Your stem cells engrafted last night. You got a count of nearly one thousand. That's real, real good."

Oh, beloved one! Be alive in me. Stay and attend this miracle of rebirth to your liking, this labor of love. I want to live! Hunt at dawn within the landscape of your sacred heart.

Flooded with phone calls this morning, my youngest brother's wedding is this afternoon and family members are calling to fill me in on the details of the gathering. I relay the good news of stem cells finding their way to my marrow and my family goes to the ceremony with a keen sense of optimism on this day of blessings and unfolding future.

My speech is slightly slurred. I have trouble standing. Now that I begin my recovery, I desperately need to leave this room. All I can think about is returning to my little house in the woods. The sky, fresh air and greenery are what I crave. The interior of my mouth is a wasteland. My face and arms are swollen up with retention of IV fluids and drugs. My skin is ruined. But I'm tremulous with the fortune of new life. With the help of excellent nurses I've come through the treatment very well. No high fevers or secondary respiratory infections have hindered me.

While most of the family attends my brother's wedding, my friend Maureen is with me today. A teacher and a traveler, she values experience second only to loyal love. Her bravery is something I continually admire and rely on. Today she is my samurai; she has come to be strong for me. It is a sacrifice as she has no appetite for illness. Her mother and grandmother have died of cancer and a beloved sister has died prematurely as well. Despite these consecutive losses, she is here, staring the nurses down, using the steel of her losses to sustain her.

I sleep most of the day but wake periodically to find her silently guarding me. After a night of literal rebirth, I enter a new infancy of sacredness and she unflinchingly guarantees me my rest. Years from now she will confide in me the moment she learned of my cancer. Traveling, alone in a hotel room, she wept and made an enraged vow that Death would not have me, too, having already exceeded his share in her sphere. No fortune is greater than this kind of love.

DECEMBER 21

The oncologist I was assigned to at the medical center is on vacation and her colleague periodically looks in on me. I am expecting to leave in three days but he has come to discuss stool samples of mine that have revealed the presence of bacteria, necessitating treatment with more strong drugs. He tells me sternly, that I will not leave the hospital until the infection is under control. I'm given Flagyl and spend the next day and a half in a violent stupor of nausea and vomiting.

My release date from the hospital recedes within the complexity of the secondary infection. The event unfolds like a dream, one in which your timing is slow, powerless, all action snowballing behind you, never getting where you're going, until you wake yourself, sweating, shouting or in tears. My mood plummets. Oh, God, what must it be like to know you will never leave the hospital.

I reach for my books and with my eyes finger bits of literature like prayer beads. But handling the weight of a book is challenging. My eyes won't focus well enough to read. I'm saved and revived by a visit from my sister and brother-in-law. I request to be read a poem by Rilke in which he describes the gifts of Orpheus. John reads the poem to me first in its native German and again in translation. It is a favorite poem, prayers with which to guide myself back from the dimming shores of end-time.

Brother Knight

Brendan comes through the door, straight from work. After a long drive in freeway traffic my brother's body is full of nervous energy. "Hey, baby! How's it shakin'." Bending near me, he gives the gift of a big sweet smile. He's gone to great lengths to remain healthy during the winter flu season so that he can visit me often in isolation. Since I was diagnosed, he has taken an active look at my household needs and finances. His generosity is nearly overwhelming to me, so much so that we speak of it. I tell him how difficult I find it to receive love and support. I try to explain why I'm so clumsy and ungracious, so quick to refuse help. I tell him that the use I will make of the cancer is to recreate my faith in abundance. We two cynics agree our faith in the goodness of life is something we will work on together.

Our long phone calls at night, preceding the transplant, have been a safety zone of sibling love and understanding. Trading insight after insight, these conversations comfort me in ways impossible to calculate. When we talk like this, I often sense his intelligence and imagination working in tandem against his own fear of cancer, of a life snatched too early before creative satisfaction, that promise of the muse, is realized. At the same time, he takes this dual energy of fear and hope and encircles me with his will. My brother never, ever falters in the belief that I will get well and I rely on the force of his convictions.

As we sit visiting, a nurse enters the room and announces that she has come to remove the Hickman port from my chest in anticipation

117

of my departure. As she announces the procedure, my whole body goes rigid. Fortunately, the attending nurse is one I like very much. She busies herself preparing my chest and laying out her tray of tools.

Brendan eyeballs the arrangement of sharp, shiny instruments. His foil is humor, his great gift. He brings his infamous wit to bear on conversation in which he and the nurse joke and laugh. From his chair, he leans on the hospital bed and holds my hand. He has a bird's-eye view of the cutting and snipping of my flesh. The nurse works purposefully and delicately. The pain is bearable, then lousy. But Bren is there and I can squeeze his hand as hard as I like and he lets me wince and tear up without skipping a beat in the dialogue, showing me how to be brave. He is articulate, like Romeo's Mercutio dying in the square making a pun of his own death. When I grip his hand hard, he lifts and kisses mine, seamlessly focused on balancing the nurse's surgery, my ability to cope and the punch line of his story. I can rest in this triad of courageous mindfulness and the nurse finishes her difficult work with a light heart.

Night Nurse

The Flagyl medication I have been given for the bacterial infection refuses to remain inside me, weakened as I am already. Its unforgiving characteristics promote acute bouts of nausea in which the slightest movement of my body sets off wave after teeth-grinding wave of it. I swallow the pills, only to have them exit my body with the merciless energy of suicide jumpers determined not to stay.

I have been vomiting on and off all day. I stumble to the bathroom at 2 AM, my entire body convulsed in dramatic heaves. I can't stop this undulation, this incoherent arching. As I hug the toilet, the minutes elude each other. I begin to gasp for breath, wild, wretched sputtering. Sliding on my knees, I pull the emergency cord and then get back to drowning at sea.

I hear her voice. She calls out, "Hold on! I'll be right back." God only knows what is going on in other isolation rooms. Suddenly, she is squatting behind me. She lays her hands on my back and begins to move them in long swirls, crossing and recrossing hands. Softly, her voice repeats a stream of phrases. "It's all right. It's all right now. Breathe. Breathe. That's it. All right. It's all right now." As the convulsions slow, I become aware of my surroundings and lean back. She lays me across her lap, ignoring the putrid fumes and the condition of my gown. She smiles at me. I tell her, "Oh, Chris, I couldn't breathe." She says, "It'll be OK now?"

She washes me off, changes my gown and carries me to the bed like a child. She sighs and tells me that since I've vomited up the

119

Flagyl, she must administer another dose. I tell her that I can't manage it. But she insists, doctor's orders. Ten minutes later, I vomit up the pill near the side of my bed. She comes with another. I plead that there must be some other medication I can take. Can I skip a dose in order to recover myself?

She sits with me for a moment and takes my pulse. She helps me work through my hour of regret, still so nauseated I can't move my head. I refuse to take the pill one more time. She gives me an extra dose of Ativan in the hope that it will settle my stomach and help me sleep. The next day, my last day in the hospital, I know she has pleaded my case. I'm told the doctor has authorized a new drug to replace the Flagyl.

After taking the new medicine I cannot detect any side effects. When I ask why it wasn't given to me in the first place, I'm told the new pill costs the hospital six dollars apiece and Flagyl is dramatically cheaper.

Late in the morning, the doctor stops in to notify me that I'm free to depart. He looks very tired. Leaving, he offers me a stiff hug that I am grateful for. He knows how much I've wanted him to sign for my release so that I can go home for Christmas. He gives me a lovely, weary smile. Perhaps my healthy resistance to the worst effects of the transplant is a small, happy truth he can take some credit for in this high-tech Veil of Tears.

V. RECOUPING IN VALHALLA

My sister brings me her family wine for the nurses. As I wrap their gifts with holiday paper, my hands are shaky with untested strength. I'm filled with gratitude for their medical expertise. I cherish their kindness and skill. Yet, a part of me never wants to think of them or their hospital habitat again. Scrawled in wobbly lines on their thank-you cards, a fragile newness of being brings an aged strangeness to my handwriting. My script is barely legible and the ribbon bows on the bottlenecks an embarrassment of ineptitude. The nurses and I know it's what's inside that counts. Mutual respect, integrity and trust: that is how we have accomplished our work together.

I lie back to rest, exhausted, and allow my obvious and profound frailty to sink in. The recognition of my own physical limitations prompts a siege of tears and self-pity. I listen for the Virgin and hearing no footsteps, I foster this moment of grief for all the trouble that has befallen me.

I feel keenly aware of a sense of fulfillment intermingled with foreboding of what the future will bring. I have more time to live! Whether I am more deserving or undeserving of this reprieve is the type of question I no longer ask myself. Whatever happens, I know it will not be measured by goodness or regret. Instead I query the universe, who will I be? How long will I last? What is my path now, having inhaled the scent of all origins in the sea-salted suspiration of Death?

I slowly shuffle around my room, packing my few belongings. The sensation of distant planets that greeted me the first time I entered this room overtakes me again, but this time, the feelings are reversed. Now, it's home that reads like a new chapter.

By the time my brother arrives with the requisite wheelchair, I'm shaking with expectation. Outside the hospital doors, I encounter a few forlorn, hunched and bundled male patients in wheelchairs, puffing on cigarettes. Posted like sentries, unnoticed, they observe the crowd of preoccupied visitors streaming through the hospital entrance. As each one inhales smoke into his ravaged frame, his eyes connect to mine in silent commentary. I too feel alien, ill, removed from the concerns of normal routine. In them I recognize the distance I've traveled.

The burden of my next task is to secede from the caregivers and find a new center for my life. I turn my face to the warmth of the sun and fresh air off the bay, hobble from the wheelchair and settle myself in the upholstered chariot from home. Can I accept a brutal realism? How many years I've already lived with a narrow apperception of possible truths. I'm going to grieve what I believed was not possible for me. Escaped for now, I'm going to stumble around in the stones of my own truths and fate will find me there.

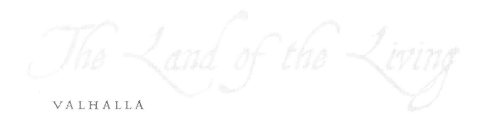

VALHALLA

Magic is afoot on Christmas morning. I hear the hushed sound of my niece and nephews' voices amidst the rustle of paper, Alex's sweet and delighted ebullience, "Just what I wanted." He and Helen appear at the side of my bed, curious and helpful. They inquire what hot beverage my sister might prepare for me downstairs and describe their favorite gifts.

A home hospice nurse arrives at the house around 10 AM. She hooks me to a rolling IV rack. Despite my appreciation of a home nurse on Christmas morning, the intrusion of more needles, more prodding, more medicine, is barely tolerable. I've had my share. I've made my escape. The work of the nurse sobers the holiday merriment and the serious observations of the children make me sad. I yearn for completion and hate distressing them with my shocking vulnerability.

The smell of freshly ground coffee I can't drink, the delicious aroma of the Christmas dinner turned to noxious roughage on my pallet, my barely mobile energy and ghastly appearance all conspire against my freedom. I want to feel good, normal, so badly. I sit at the holiday dinner table for as long as I can, then curl up in a blanket on the rug in front of the fire. I lie there, close my eyes and give thanks like a person rescued who reveres the wholesome activity of the saviors.

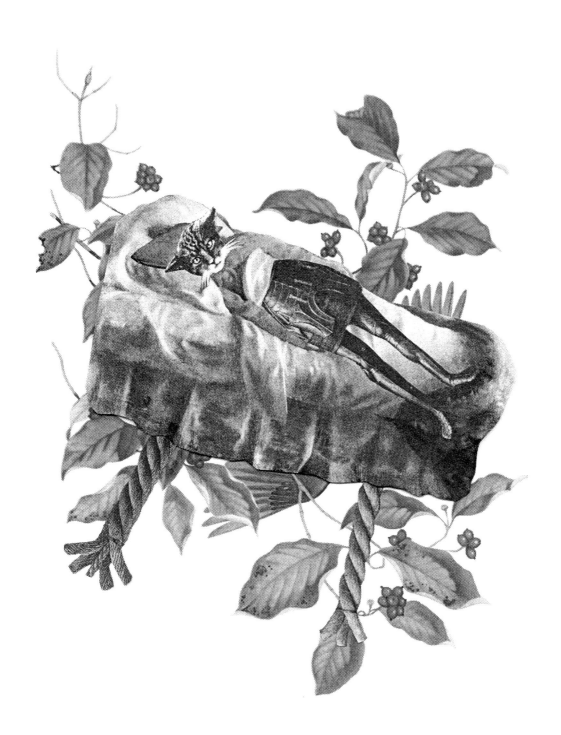

The frightening weakness that occupies my body does not improve and I sleep on and off during the days preceding the New Year. I come downstairs to the kitchen for half-hour visits only. I'm still suffering the last effects of the intestinal disorder contracted in the hospital, still painfully exuding the waste of chemical poisons. Salves for my skin and copious amounts of licorice tea to sooth my mucous membrane help. Each meal is a major experiment. I fear that nothing will ever taste good again.

I left the hospital riding on the back of my hope, like a woman in a parade waving reassuringly to the crowd. I tried not to suspect that recovery might unfold as a long and rigorous trial. But patience has never been my strong suit, and the impatience I feel now to recover grates at my nerves and trespasses on my happiness. I'm alive; never mind the fear and discomfort. Yet my mind is unsteady, traumatized. I've read that infants in the first few months of life cry on awakening from sleep because they dream of their life in the womb, remembering the trauma of birth each time they wake.

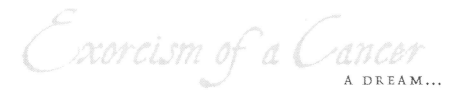

I

ON THE THIRD DAY OUT

i dream of *the hospital wing but the features of the isolation room are condensed in an airless, one-dimensional collage of overlapping esthetics. My hospital bed is cranked up high off the floor where I lie amongst starched pillows. A highly agitated physician rushes in, white coattails flying and papers billowing off his clipboard. He shouts that doctors have just failed to resuscitate an impostor of Jesus Christ.*

I'm silenced by the power of association. Is the physician mad or is it true? Was the patient a charlatan or has Christ returned, unrecognized, and died again? It's better they have not saved him. What would we have done with a brain-dead Jesus? The doctor tells me that the impostor was a bum who had "plagued them over the years." Just before he died, they were able to obtain a stool sample as proof of his deception. He shows me a board smudged with labeled excrements. He points to the type obtained from the transient.

As he does this, the vision of a small man, perhaps four feet high, appears before me from a mist. He wears an old-fashioned detective's trench coat. The large, stand-up collar frames a backdrop for his head. The coat drags behind his worn-out shoes and his heavy cuffs hang below his hands.

All that can be seen of his body is a patch of face. His jaundiced complexion is framed by wiry, ill-kept hair. Frizzy strands jut from underneath a brown, wide-brimmed wool fedora.

His eyes are black with tiny white reflections of light at the center. His nose is sharp. His coated teeth are scummy with flecks of brown and yellow. He personifies disease in a troubling, rodent-like caricature, whose shuffling gait conjures an unhealthy dust. When he looks at me, I see that he has no soul.

II

in the shifting *dream light, I now inhabit the stylized setting of a fifties magazine advertisement. Here, I am a young girl being led by a woman from a mansion to an expensive vintage automobile. She wears a full-skirted, emerald-green crinoline dress, paired with expensive costume jewelry. She strikes model-like poses in high heels as she attempts to drag me, struggling, to the car.*

Once inside, she turns to me, transformed. Thickly dwarfed with age and sunken into the driver's seat, she is silent and sluggish. Her thinning hair is gray and dull against a heavily powdered face. Under her nose, her lipstick is smeared in exaggerated peaks of glistening pink. She stares straight ahead, sucks her lips and refuses to acknowledge me. I recognize her as the mother of a woman who was my eighth-grade teacher and who is now being treated for a recurrence of breast cancer. I worry whether my teacher's mother will be able to drive our car.

Suddenly, I acknowledge an invisible evil floating above the back seats. I identify the disembodied vapor as the little diseased man, the rat with no soul. Frantically, I scream and shout at the Mother to help me, but still mute, she plays chauffeur to the demon. In desperation, I unwind a lever in the ceiling of the car, opening a screened vent. With my face horribly contorted, I scream in threes, "I cast thee out. I cast thee out. I cast thee out." Like a cartoon tornado, the vapor swirls around the interior of the car and vanishes through the metal mesh.

I announce our salvation to the Mother. I'm furious with her. I tell her I can prove the existence of the evil visitor. I roll down the window of the car and pull a dismembered leg from the vanishing highway. I rest it on the seat between us. Still silent, she only glances at the bloody stump.

*Already
my escape preoccupies me. I'm not entirely able to believe in it. A
wild animal rushing from an opened cage, I look back to interpret what force
has restrained me and sense that my freedom is simply a new dimension whose limits I do not yet understand. The trick is not considering anything but the moment. I
savor and reinterpret all familiar things. When my brother-in-law takes me through
the woods to walk in the nearby vineyard, it isn't just a morning stroll, but the
first walk in nature of my new life. What I see on the mountain are my first tree-
fringed winter skies, my first sight of pond water ringed by emerald grass, the
grapevines all canes and skeletal leaves. The air is cold and stringent, infused
with the smell of well-drained soil. John's arm bearing my weight, I'm weak
and struggle for breath. I am euphoric.*

My sister, her husband and
their children are classical music aficionados. They're passionate about
chamber music and opera, in particular Wagner's opera, *The Ring*. In
good humor, they refer to their home in the woods as Valhalla.
Throughout my cancer treatments, reference was made to me here as
Brunhild.

My sister devotes herself to me in my period of stem-cell recovery as she did during all my cancer treatments, making room for my
trouble in her life unhesitatingly. She fills in any and all gaps in my
care that she can find. She mothers me and moves in my life as a no-
nonsense guide helping me to consider the practical aspects of my
situation: wig or no wig, the leave of absence from my job, my

finances. She brings her intelligence and formidable pursuit of accuracy to garner information on cancer and its treatment. Though we live very separate lives, in this time of illness I am irrevocably reminded that any feeling of distance between us is merely a habit of perception, grounded in our difficult childhood.

This exhausting holiday week through New Year's, she and my brother-in-law have given me their bed and sleep on their living-room floor in front of the fire. My sister keeps a borrowed baby intercom on a side table so that she can detect any change in my breathing or hear me if I call. In unpleasant moments of frustration, sadness and menacing dreams, she offers me reassurance and her confidence in my recovery.

In the dead of night
I wake to find my sister
sitting on the side of the bed. My
restless sounds through the intercom
have summoned her. I see her beautiful face,
half illuminated from a distance by lamplight. Her
long hair trails down her back. I never see her with it
down. Whispering in the dark, in her plaid nightgown, it is as
though no years have passed since we were young. She observes me
closely and asks softly, "Are you OK?" So comforting is her presence that I
reach out and hold onto her arm so that she will never leave me. In simple sen-
tences and small acts of affection, we allude to the love alive in our hearts. We bridge the
tempered past, filled with what we cannot undo or understand about each other.

Maggy and John have long been planning a New Year's Eve party and a piano concert to be performed by a close friend whose book on Beethoven's life and music has just been published to much scholarly acclaim. As Bill practices Beethoven's Opus 111 for tonight's performance, I watch him from beneath my comforter on the couch. As he plays, he slow-dances, closes his eyes and listens, understanding and interpreting the composition with each finger of his hands. He moves to the music as though soul-feeding, a perfect blend of emotion, skill and intellect rising toward what is divine. As I listen here or from the bed upstairs, he is the perfect companion, a detached and unassuming channel of artfulness.

I feel blessed to witness his dedication, as though the music had been arranged, timed, especially for my purpose. In the presence of the Muse, I recognize the arrival of a deep-seeded blossoming of my own creativity, the awareness of which brings me repeatedly to tears. I don't attempt to understand what is coming; it has no agenda or strategy. Bill's manifestation of impassioned discipline activates a renewed purpose to emanate my own bliss, to follow nothing but the sound of an inner rhapsody for as long as I can.

In contrast to moments of spiritual clarity, I remain frightened by post-transplant side effects. The medical authorities parrot the haunting phrase "side effects are highly variable." In other words, they have no idea what the lasting complications will be. Each body responds differently. The metallic taste on my tongue, reminding me of Comet and Clorox, gradually registers food as the flavorless texture of cat fur, the dull taste of cardboard, and, next, a faint fruitiness, as though I snacked on candy wrappers. Finally, I attain actual and glorious flavors.

My sense of smell is remarkably dimmed. Not being able to smell is like seeing a pooh-pooh pillow release its air without a sound. It's just not the same fun. However, I only really notice this when others around me are complaining of smelly socks, garlic or other impolite odors. I suffer a pronounced numbness of the skin on my back, still triggering the analogy of dead parts in my psyche. In fact, my skin *is* dying off, as well as my fingernails and toenails, which loosen themselves and grow increasingly discolored each day. Pushing upward at the base of the cuticle, rippled and pearly claws emerge. I've started praying for hair.

Brought to my bedside, my beloved dog, Josephine, visibly sulks when she finally sees me. I believe she assumes that I have forsaken her this long while, favoring my sister's house and company. I yearn for my little home in the woods with her, my lofty nest with a view. My family conspires against my independent streak, thinking me foolish to return there unaccompanied after only two weeks. I resolve this conflict by inviting my mom to come for a few days and encouraging visits from friends.

JANUARY 10, 1995

Maggy drives me to my first oncology appointment since late November, when my oncologist took a core sample of my bone marrow preceding the transplant. It is my first major outing since being released from the hospital and my energy fades quickly. We wait a long time in the lobby until my sister informs the receptionist of my weakening condition. A nurse ushers us into a room, where we continue to wait.

When my oncologist walks through the open door he observes me with measured thoughtfulness. For the first time since I've known him he does not smile or meet my eyes with a direct gaze. I have anticipated a commemorative mood. Perhaps he is having a bad day, hence the wait, or he feels a culpable remorse on witnessing the devastation of my physical appearance, or both.

He squats by my chair and looks down at the floor while we speak. I want to reassure him, yet, at the same time, let him look at what the drugs have done. Be with me in the good times and the bad. Perhaps a patient who fought a more difficult fight than mine has died today, or a young person he wanted with all his skill and heart to live did not. I do not ask him how he feels about what I have gone through on his recommendation. Nor do I ask him how he copes with the responsibility of his recommendations. I do not judge him, because his belief in my recovery makes our bond a strong one. I love him for his ability to hope and for choosing me to believe in. I will always remember my moments with him and his vision of my cure. In time, I may be for him a grim footnote or a statistical point of rejoicing. If my medical coverage changes, I might lose all sight of him and his belief in my recovery. Is there room amidst the industry of cancer for affection, friendship or approval? Some days yes, yes! Not today, in this too, too busy oncology office.

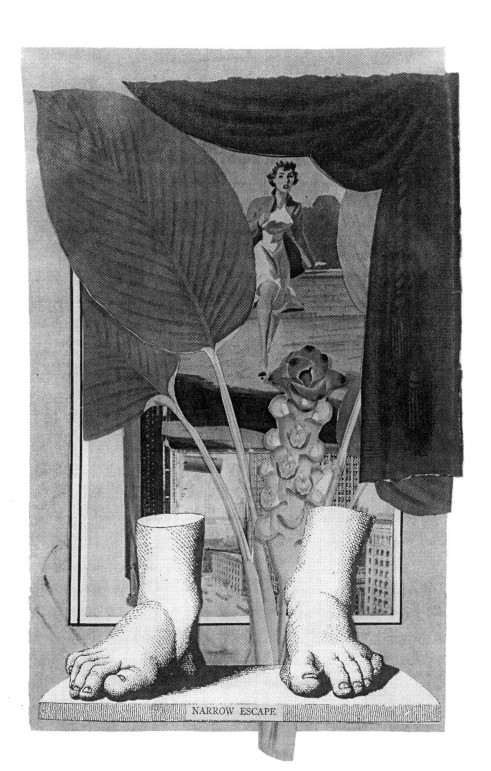

NARROW ESCAPE

My younger brother, Gavin, arrives for a visit. He comes because I ask him for his help in a ritual. With him he brings his little smoke, Indian sage in a bundle, to perform a cleansing of my house, my garden and myself. I count on his ability to penetrate the brittle, mirrored coating of reality. I have not seen much of him because he conspicuously absences himself from my medical drama for his own reasons, entering and exiting at crucial junctures only. I've missed him and felt hurt by his reserve, feeling at the same time vastly supported by others and concerned that his dread for me goes uncomforted by the family. I understand how painful it is to think of losing one another. During this troubled time, he has concentrated on his own life and aspires for a family of his own. In autumn of last year, I was happy to learn from him that he has fallen deeply in love. In a few short months, during my time in isolation, he married. He yearns, very much, for a child.

My brother, a poet and musician, is the most intuitive and emotional person I know. He pays attention to how life feels. With his smoking wand of sage, he walks through the house and garden, refreshing dismal corners and cleansing the air of the last stale breath of illness. Along the stone steps of the garden he senses the sigh of my once beloved, still echoing a last adieu. In the garden, amongst budding roses, he approaches my deserted shrine. I have not told him of my struggles with the Virgin. He becomes thoughtful, serious. He turns and asks me, "What happened here? Why have you abandoned this place?" After hearing my story, he is quiet. He waits for his intuition to speak to him. Finally, after a long silence, he says, "Bec, you should put a picture of yourself here, pray for yourself in front of it. Use an image that represents what your energy is now. A picture of your spirit that you can give thanks for."

When my brother says this, I immediately know which image he has tapped into. A week ago I painted an abstract portrait of my body energy, a chakra-based image I'm extremely drawn to. I take my brother's advice and recreate a likeness of it in the alcove of the shrine. As I fill the dish pond in its center with clean water, I think of my brother and his gift of perception. From my bench, I observe the garden dwellers, bees, dragonflies, birds and lizards, dip and drink in the belly of the shrine. All they need surrounds them.

When I see Gavin next, our families are all together to celebrate his wedding now that I'm strong enough to attend a party. He puts a steady hand on my shoulder and smiles into my eyes, inspects my bald head for new hair. Between us there is abundant reverence. He says, "Well, did you put your picture up? Good, I'm so glad." He leads me to the couch, telling me that he has someone I need to meet: Harry, his wife's brother, a person who reminds him of me.

VI. THE RESURRECTION OF DELIGHT

Slowly, I'm summoning the courage to leave my job in favor of something less demanding of my resources. I attend a meeting of fellow managers and hope for a chance to discuss working part-time with my employer. I am the only woman present. In the managerial atmosphere of the group meeting, my professional ego rises to engage in competitive discussion. My old habits of jockeying for mental dominance and approval float to the surface, then quickly pass away again.

Startled by the impasse, I recognize in stark and rudimentary terms that the use of this energy no longer serves me. I think to myself, why do I care so much about having to be right or best, such sterile desires? I will forfeit my hard-won power and be replaced. And piece by piece, our identities, these relationships, this business, will all be fondly relegated to the past. There, each and every one of us will be picked over by the passing vagrant of memory. I grasp hold of the anxiety I feel and set it aside like a favorite cup so cracked and worn it will no longer hold water. I sit back and take a deep breath in the light of a subtler life.

I

I arrive at my first radiology appointment slightly apprehensive. I expect to be unpopular with the technicians because I have steadfastly rejected the tattooing procedure. I don't want to be reminded of this treatment every time I look at my breasts for the rest of my natural life. I'm just too young for that. Radiologists favor tattooing the skin. They create a permanent site map on the body to insure the accuracy of the radiation. There is nothing decorative about these tattoos, just the blunt marks of latitude and longitude.

The radiology technicians are irritated with me for denying them their protocol. Their white coats in the darkened room rustle with each measurement as they draw on my breast and ribs in indelible ink. Indignantly and condescendingly, they lecture me about the hazards of blurred lines. I am quietly determined and assure them that I will guard their work carefully.

In the mirror of the radiology dressing room, blue ink against my white skin imitates the butcher's line left on a haunch of meat. Numbered flesh. I decide to leave my hat behind. It seems absurd to wear a hat to a shirtless, indoor event.

I emerge from the changing room, hairless, with only droplet earrings to frame my face. The handsome, manly technician guides me to the radiation room. Most of his patients are elderly. We are roughly the

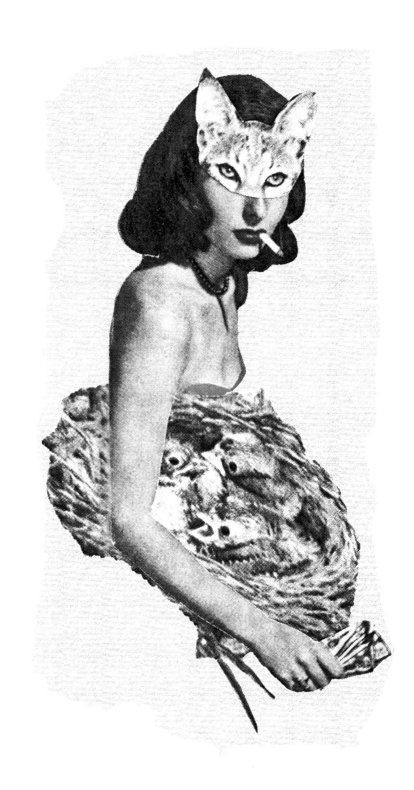

same age and my youth unnerves him. He offers a kind smile and with a flickering gleam in his eye he says, "You know, you look good bald." Glowing in more ways than one, I end up flirting my way through the twenty-six sessions of radiation, the only opportunity I have to take my shirt off for a guy.

II

In the lobby of the gynecologist's office I stare at my dead, rippled fingernails. Pushed upward by new pink growth at the cuticles, my old nails arch painfully forward, discolored, the last assault of chemo drugs exiting my body. I have dutifully come for my annual exam despite my current aversion to yet more scrutiny by doctors. My radiated breast chafes against my blouse.

From the moment my gynecologist greets me, she makes it clear that she's monitored the course of my treatments and that the prospect of cancer and chemotherapy is appalling to her. She subtly keeps her physical distance as though a tumor might leap from me and attach itself to her neck or scalp, embed itself there like a brooding tick.

I'm having trouble concentrating because her fear distracts me. It's difficult to appreciate her words when she tells me how brave she thinks I am and how she admires my ability to choose such a difficult path. The exam proves unexpectedly painful. I suspect my mucous membrane and hormone balance, stripped and devastated by the transplant, is the cause. I have never had an abnormal Pap smear.

143

Days later I find a message from her on my tape machine. In a voice full of foreboding, she commands me to see her; the result of my test is of grave concern. In her office, she explains that my Pap smear has revealed an alarming evidence of irregular tissue. She is fairly certain that I have cervical cancer.

As I listen to her rationale, I hear the sound of flipping switches on a panel of garish stage lights. I wrap my body in a dramatic flood of cornball illumination. Her words bounce off me, unable to penetrate its powerful glow. In a firm voice I suggest the possibility that the bone-marrow transplant might be the cause of abnormal tissue, but she fails to calm herself and she insists I see my oncologist immediately. I look into her face and know fear and concern cloud her perception of me. She perceives me as vulnerable to new tumors and I cannot trust her judgment. The one thing I know I must do is get away from her opinion immediately.

A new gynecologist examines me and, after speaking with my oncologist, confirms my own suspicions. The severity of hormonal disruption caused by my treatments, combined with a loss of mucous membrane, has seared the tissue of my vaginal wall. Like pan-fried flesh, it bleeds when stuck. After the second exam, my fragile tissues open in long paper cuts at the slightest friction. Will this too pass? Estrogen is not an option.

Journeying Toward Euphoria

I

I begin a new series of artwork in my studio. Years have past since my last undisturbed period for artistic expression. The weather is cold and wet. Winter storms sweep across the face of the mountain and the studio is damp and smelly with the faint scent of kerosene. Consistent energy comes and goes like an unreliable friend but my creative spirit is irrepressible. It bounds and leaps forward, frisks in all directions full of unpredictable ambitions and emotions. I have to challenge myself to work fast enough to capture all that I envision in paper Assemblage. It's all about staying out of the way, letting go of expectation in life and art, bowing to the energy of the Muse, the mothering marrow birthing itself in my blood.

I hang thirty-two pieces of work in a local gallery space and all of them sell at the opening. This is a triumph I can hardly contain. The images, hanging in a narrow room, assemble themselves like stations of the cross, speak like witnesses to the stages and states of mind I have inhabited in the past year. The images tell their own stories, endowed with their own power, some sadly poignant, others tragic or funny, erotic or spiritual. I realize that the open and intimate images that have come through me speak to others in a universal way. Moved by the poetic liner notes I've written for each artwork, patrons and friends strongly suggest that I expand the writing into a book.

What
say I to the stream? Waiting, stopping to talk is not its nature.
Listening to my tape deck, I am inside the music and dance in place at my table
of paper. I dodge and weave, eluding moments of willfulness and analysis. I sing or
hum to free my mind and divert the ego from critiquing its own fiction. I combine
scraps of images, cutouts and colored paper until the imagery locks into its own place, a
psychic jigsaw that manifests a story of its own choosing, the dream story of the self.

The privately theatrical and dreamlike symbolism of figures and objects interacting
in rooms and landscapes mesmerize me, and I bend like Narcissus to the reflection of my own
psychology. Filtered through the waters and roots of my unconscious and delivered by the
hands of the Muse, I delight in the mirror of my interpretations and in defiance of
myth, find ultimate satisfaction and renewal in rumors of my soul. I value these
images as clues to the body politic, subtle messages on the health of
my mind/body, a process that feels central to my
survival.

I arrive home late, in the company of friends who have traveled to attend the opening. I am in heaven. Exhilarated, like a whistling teakettle, I talk and laugh, so happy to be alive. From the patio I lead two friends down the steep, unlit flagstone steps. Stupidly invincible in party shoes, I carry bedding to a spare room in my neighbor's house below. Paul jokes from the top of the stairs and we turn to laugh. Our eyes blinded by the patio lights we see his gesturing frame as a backlit silhouette. My next step down finds me literally floating on air. To the horror of my friends, I am bruised but undamaged after rolling down a half dozen sharp-edged steps, landing in leaf duff at the base of a tree. Afterward, in the quiet house, I put ice on my thigh and, smiling, realize that I've fallen back to Earth, on my swollen hip a little bruise of silver cloud.

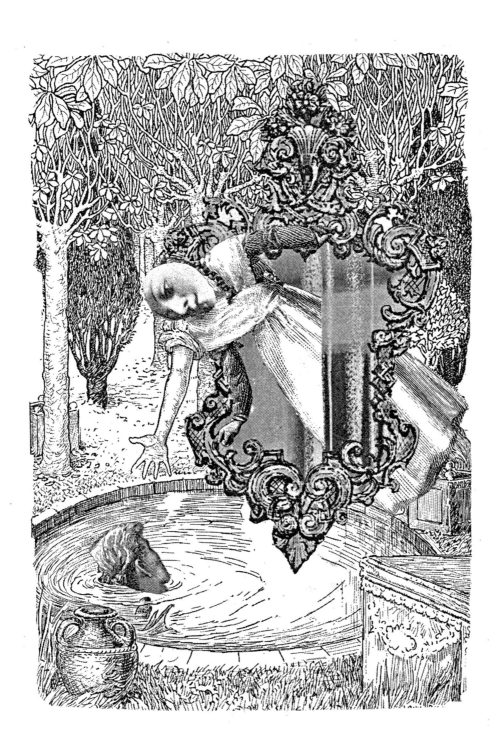

II

I make a practice of dancing alone every day or whenever I can. I ritualize the dancing with poetic movement that connects me with my body, frees my spirit and dominates a terror of tumors. Music of Deep Forest, Ensemble Alcatraz, music of Mali, Nigeria and Tanzania, Italian folk songs, Japanese Khotto, French medieval court music, Tuva and pygmy singers, flamenco, blues, gypsy jazz and opera soloists, music full of singing, moods and rhythm. Dancing, my battle to physically stabilize becomes literal, a narrative of movements, life and death matters acted out in emotional and energetic dance, critical to health. My body tells the story of its bones and blood, grief and exaltation. Dancing is my singular purgative, a medicine that expels the chemical confusion sullying my physiology. Moving to music gracefully calms me and placates the corked rage of calamity. No one has spoken to me about the experience of chemical menopause. It has never been mentioned. I notice it first when dancing, a periodic sluggishness lurking in the background, a whiff of despair in the mood. But I take those and other fears and make them holy. Now, it's only when dancing that I sense the presence of the Divine.

As

I dance I visualize my insides,

an immense interior full of visceral imagery,

my organs and muscle, tissue and bone healthy and

whole. Gradually, as I sway to poignant singing, my exterior

shape emerges, a heavily bordered outline full of nightscape packed

with dense nebula of stars. Twirling in large circles I imagine whirling,

loosely binding myself in golden thread, spun like tawny honey, then melting into

a pool of creamy light. My face is wet with tears. I sense the presence of witnesses,

and then her arm, extended downward above me, fingers tightly gripping the top of my

head. One violent twist is all it will take, her face benevolent, close to mine. She has

not visited for a long while but I know what she is there to show me that life and

death, divinity and suffering, are inseparable, inevitable. I do not decide when or why

I will die. My knees crumple and I sit heavily onto the floor in distress. Why

must it be this way? I don't want to accept it. Let me believe what I think

and feel makes a difference to disease, allow the brilliance of living to

outshine Death for a little while.

A DREAM...

i wait in *the indigo light of predawn in a desert terrain I hold dear, a familiar place ringed with austere and toothy shapes of barren mountains. In the night the distant rock perimeter densely black as the air is blue.*

I have come here with four elderly men. We are shy friends, a younger woman amongst Indian compañeros. As a frosty wind sweeps the desert floor, we wait together in anticipation of a definitive moment. We speak sparingly in hushed, animated tones. The phosphorescence of their white muslin clothes illuminates our bodies. They stand slouched, shoulder to shoulder, smoking and tapping their feet to keep warm. They stare at the ground in the middle of our circle and their golden faces glow as though lit by the flames of a fire.

As the men acknowledge an exact calibration of shifting light, a discreet turbulence moves through them. With abrupt nods of their heads, smiling and blinking their eyes, they shoo me from our congregation with their hands. I stride away from them, amongst the dim shapes of desert occupants. The vibration of each of my steps brings light and quickens the hue of morning. Each time I turn and wave, they raise their arms from beneath serapes and gesture. In no time, their figures become one with the shadows.

I walk with resolution, alert in the absence of desire. Nearer the mountain, I come upon an unending horizontal cylinder of wind, a supernatural stream four feet across and suspended in the larger air three feet above the ground. The exterior velocity of the air forms a translucent tunnel, a vacuum of air where thousands of differing seeds are blown to a further destiny.

I penetrate the sacred conduit, step into its fertile path and stay. Seeds ping and thud against me, rest in rivulets on my outstretched arms. I quiet all my questions, and then peacefully salute the cresting sun as it reveals the day.

The men greet my return with ceremony, their eyes resplendent as they hold their hats in their hands, nod, and tenderly pat my back with affection. They congratulate me with the music of gentle laughter, "Amiga. Bueno. You have done well."

VII. THE INVOLUTION OF BELIEF

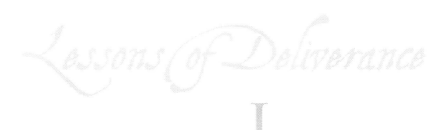

Lessons of Deliverance

I

And now...the devoted, benevolent faces turn away to fresh concerns. The battle has been won. I stand detached in a different field, the commonplace, and watch the petty, fettered events of life creep in. Is it selfish to yearn for the precious honey of love in huge dollops, buckets full, oceans of affection? Were we not meant for this?

Sisters, stay, why not sit for hours to brush each other's hair and sing together at dusk? Brothers, why wait inside and worry, walk with me amongst the trees again and make a sonnet of your life? Relinquish me not to the ponderous task of beginning again, alone, the small and tedious obligations of life. Keep me with you. Wedge yourselves between the rocks of all my fears.

II

I detach myself from my job with a last special event and wine auction. The effort it takes and success it brings leaves me guiltless and ready to go. With new eyes I travel around for a possible last look at the world. I visit Maine and the sea. In summer, I go northeast to a river, then north to a woodland lake. I'm well loved by dear friends in all these places.

With my father and brothers, I pack into the southern Sierras to rest by the water of cirques. At 7,000 feet, in a thinning tree line, I pick a few sage leaves for drying and burning. In a meadow, an elaborate architecture of cut grass forms the four-foot dome of a rodent's house. As I kneel to wash my face, a slender snake floats by, momentarily adrift in snow-melted amber creek water. Breaking through trees into my silence, a curious doe lingers to look me in the eye. These gifts of grace are what I've come for, most holy mountain temples not lost to me. Through them I find my place in the world. At this altitude, my mind is clear and filled with peaceful gratitude. Being here in the mountains again appeases the stormy weather of regret I sometimes feel.

I determine to say goodbye to a friend who is within days of dying and visit her on the way to my first biannual checkup. I brace myself to face both the specter of death and the results of my tumor-marker blood tests all in the same morning. My friend's recurrence of breast cancer has been unexpected, swift and fatal. Ten years ago I was the caretaker on her ranch, where we worked together soon after her first mastectomy.

Her daughter greets me at the door and invites me to visit her room. Entering its shuttered interior, I catch sight of my altered friend, propped up in bed, studying things not visible to me. I understand from her manner that she is still readying herself for death and is not quite ready to go. She is still finding meaning, reflecting and remembering. I hesitate before approaching and for thirty seconds imagine my own death, that it be free of agony.

I sit by the bed, take her hand and let her know I am there. She recognizes me instantly and repeatedly attempts to communicate in fragmented two-word sentences. For terminal pain, the hospice nurse has given my friend a gift, a generous dose of morphine that eases her suffering but affects her ability to form words. She attempts, gracious as always, to explain her efforts to keep track of my illness and how thrilled she is that I'm recovering so well. I cannot understand most of what she says, but this matters very little to our conversation. Though her words are incoherent, her face expresses the sweetness of better days and her fond memories of the period of her history we spent together. Suddenly, she stops her bewildering attempt at normal conversation and closes her eyes in gathering concentration. I sit with her silently for long last moments and move to go. Finally, she relies on a simple message to describe what she is living out past all tragedy and regret. Turning her head on the pillow, she looks me straight in the eye, squeezes my hand and says in a clear and dulcet voice, "Love. Love. So much love."

IV

In the throes of chemical menopause I no longer hear the voice of the Friend, and I mistrust the unpredictable love and presence of the Virgin. To love her is to love and accept myself wholly, something I am afraid to do. Instead, I strive to fall in love, a drought-stricken tree laden in blossoms, every gene sending my message to the bees. In this climacteric phase, I write desperately long-winded affirmations to encourage the arrival of an ideal mate. I wear tight-fitting sweaters to the grocery store and while standing in line imagine myself kissing attractive strangers. In the death of menses, I review my missed opportunities to bear and birth, motherhood forfeited forever in this life. Now I'm stripped of my own estrogen and am forbidden substitutes, no allies to keep the she-wolves of change away.

My ovaries harmonize in diminishing song, sirens lilting and clashing in E minor. They strain their fading voices toward Odysseus, lost off the coast of Circe's island. In this hormonal enchantment, my last restige of maidenhood pales to a colorless form. I have become a woman, full-bodied, and the shy, lithe girl of my past slips forever from me.

Erotic tension heightens desire. Yet...naked in the sleepless night, sweating, soaked by flashes in the sable of holy darkness, it is only you, Mother of all mothers, your essence that I feel near me. But, sweetest of all friends, I fear the gruesome sovereignty of your gentle hand. I only dare to live at a distance from the perfumed flower of your being. It is here, in our cloistered dimension, with you and I orbiting together between waking and dreaming, that I call to my elusive, earthly lover. Lover, lover, bend near me and drop your fruit-filled branches.

157

The austerity of spiritual experience and the euphoria of escape, spiked with a terror of premature death, join in me and interact in an oscillating physical urgency, mitochondria fueling the fresh marrow growing in my bones. A lascivious vitality saturates my body, filling dry holes to the brim. My need to hydrate, no matter the erroneous propagation, my need to hang on to the winged feet of departing divinity, is what defines me. I want to live. Do you hear? Fall in love once more before I die. What spell might I cast, what plea could I cry upward? Might I jam open with dry sticks the portal of the Venus gate? Give me love to hold onto; I'm too young for the company of crones. Don't let lust fade with desiccating fever, dry leaves scraping well-paved streets.

V

The anniversaries of my cancer treatment loom up and over me shake their rattles and grin with unseeing eyes. A self-pitying mood withers the edge of my composure and reaches for the quick drunk of blame. I snap and bark when bothered. A postmenstrual fury is mounting, humping around inside me. Swinging from my rib bones, it thumps and hurls itself against the hollow cavity of my chest.

I pick out my least favorite dishes from the cupboard: one mug, three saucers, a platter and a vase. Willful and resolute, my anger steers me into the yard. With all the force I can summon, I launch and smash the pottery against the brick of the garden wall. Unsatisfied, the ragged

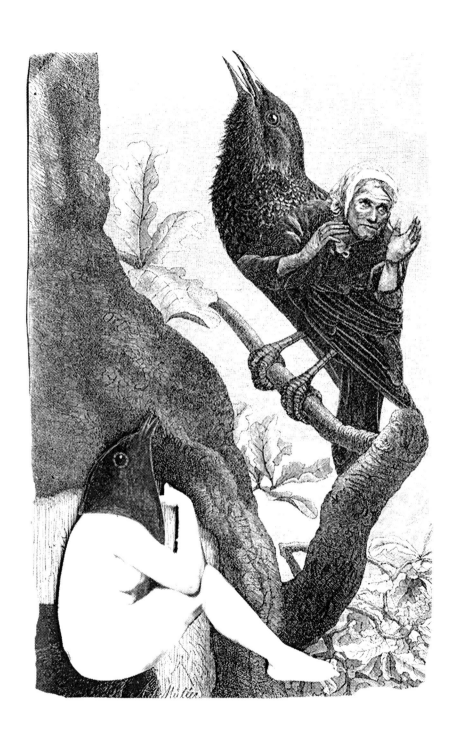

breath of frenzy overtakes me. Panting, I run to the house for cover. Entering through the back hall, I realize the solid core door of the water heater closet is an ideal baffle for my rage, this raucous celebration of misfortune.

I slam the door once, not hard enough, twice harder, three, four, five, then six times...follow me into this slamming trance. I yell obscenities to the rhythm of banging wood, and then sob *Mama, Mama*, till I slump from the heated doorknob.

Exhausted and shaken, I wash my face. When I'm ready to lift my head again, all I can think to do is dance.

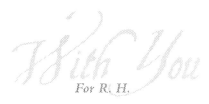

With You

For R. H.

I rely on your pact with me that no form of my anger will separate us. We will not turn away from what I say or do. My nice-girl face twists and tightens to birth a nasty, bloody-eyed snarl. I hear my own voice, a loathsome voice that chokes up words like odious minions, ripping and tearing at every feeling. Then emotion swells my expressions, weeping eyes, running nose and blotchy cheeks reducing my face to a blur of fleshy lamentation.

My braying lips are magnified, slick and shiny with tears and drool. They turn upward, a sputtering mouthpiece that protests a litany of abandonment, stale bile flooding the worn-out tracks of logic. The heat of my ire reflects off the surface of your expressive body. You send only your unwavering eyes to meet me. In them, I see the wide road ahead beyond the precipice of my narrow passage, where I jerk and flail, the pale puppet of old sorrows.

nights later i dream...*that I float down from above to see myself in a strange bed, unable to rest or sleep. Tossing and turning, I wrest the sheets fearfully in the dark. In a bright luster of moonlight I lie with my arm against my forehead in the pose of a thoughtful heroine facing certain doom. Close up, I gaze stricken into the tangled face of my own anxious narrative. The fingers of my other hand circle the scar on my breast, caress it, the way a sad ballerina breaks the heart of the audience as she enters, dancing in a spotlight, from stage left.*

You crack open the door. I sense your hushed concern. The warm glow of a well-lit house floods past your fatherly silhouette. I feel small in the bed, a child again. Here, in my dream, you draw near me. I see your resplendent face and your crescent ring of white hair. Your belly appears unusually large and round from beneath your elegant vest. Your hands rest on its ledge, protective and expectant.

Like a mother, you bend over me, stroke my hair and whisper, "Were you afraid?" You go to the window and pull back the drape. You say in your poet's voice, "Look, love, how beautiful the moon and stars." It's true. The moon appears divine, suspended close and gleaming at the sill, bathing our bodies with shimmering light. Stars gather at her shoulders in graceful boughs.

In the cool air of morning, I listen to music and dance. I realize the dream of your pregnant body when I let my belly hang full.

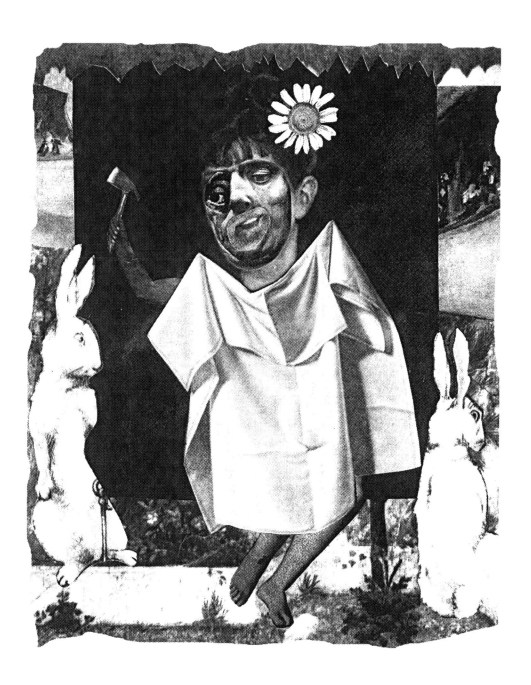

A man akin to me has crossed my path. The calm knowing of a sure thing, the mutual sense of intimacy and inevitability that accompanies the arrival of love, balances the sparks and flares of attraction between us. We have been calling for one another across a lonely void, only to have a simple gesture of our siblings unite us.

This new love diverges from my romantic vita, wherein I have loved what was not possible to possess, leaving me luxurious room for solitude. But this love takes sudden root and its vigorous tendrils surround me. The two faces of my psyche are at once content and rebellious, serene and recalcitrant, optimistic and apprehensive. Now that it's arrived, have I lived alone for too long, been too close to death to open to the simple joys, the meat and veins, sticks and stones of mated love again?

Might Persephone and Eurydice emerge, unafraid of history, to delight in the pleasures of sunlight and defy the moldering floor of eternity? Where can the physical and the spiritual unite in me? How can I muster the innocence of sexual surrender, carrying the knowledge of my own mortality? You must understand that for me now, both God and Death are everywhere. They sit, aged spectators, together, and keep a running commentary on the subject of my foibles.

Oh, Our Lady, embrace me again without hesitation. Let me bury my face between your breasts and breathe in the comfort of your compassionate being. Don't break me in two with your love. Show me how to bring this devotion earthward and lay it at the feet of a true heart.

Before me your robed body, nova suspended in the miraculous
sky of Juan Diego's watery blue-stained cloth, Guadalupe, your face
unsmiling, missing even a subtle up curve of lips. A hint of recognition at your mouth is all that betrays the witness of your solitude. The
thin plucked arches high on your brow, the comely trace of double
chin at your neck at odds with the heaviness of your down cast eyes,
one lid nearly closed as though drugged with sadness. I'm made anxious by the humble set of your clasped hands. Cupped in place,
eternally chaste, as the neckline of your dress made limp with the
damp of immutable sorrow. Your head is bowed, hardworking arms
captured in an act of perpetual pleading so dense with effort it dulls
the rays of your aura to bronze.

A stance so unlike Mary's blond radiance, arms and hands outstretched, expansive, dainty white feet perfectly balanced on her tiny
globe. Instead, at the brown curve of your unwashed ankles, a dispas-
sionate angel grips the crescent of a changeable moon, back bent with
the weight of his cumbrous burden. Common cloth blends your
human image with the washed palate of holiness, rust of water stain
and blush of dust, earth tones of gold flake and indigo, olive and stone.
In earnest prayer, I catch the scent of musk from your orgiastic release
of Castilian roses, the bright and remorseless gaiety of message that
drained the color from your sepia cheek. You gave the gift of your
vitality as evidence for the faithless, but the rainbow petal profusion
of your power was not enough. An idol proved necessary to worship.

You gave a somber transference, proof that consoles us, as one disconsolate soul recognizes another, comforted by the sad tired sweetness of your roseate prayer.

But...where lives the joyful, sensual ingénue of my visitations appearing at the apex of need, reciprocal twin that expresses maternal endearments the ceaseless adjuration of your portrait does not allow? How rises the insatiable Goddess whose violent love tutors spiritual ignorance, who, wild and shining with fluttering hands, makes a dance of blood and mutilation? From what place comes the trinity who stands in defense of fire, bright lit burning of transfiguration, swinging the two-sided blade of jubilance and suffering in arcs above her crowns?

Transfixed by the threefold unity of your aspect, a communion of humility, compassion and ferocity, I struggle with a spiritual synthesis that leads and confuses me, enlightens and confounds. When and why do you lift your head and fondly smile, oh savage animation that roams untamed by association?

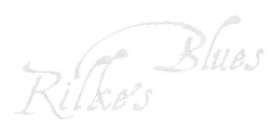

Rilke's Blues

If I could just get up every morning and shout *hallelujah, hallelujah, hallelujah*, ten or twenty times, I know I'd feel better. Even if all I could do were to whisper it, *hallelujah*, move my body in rhythm, the quicker my heart would beat. Instead, I open my eyes to a post-menses spirit, full up with longing for the past. My heart is heavy with the moment, my body graceless with concern. I say, Becca, how come you're not praising, how come you're not lifting up your arms? Fall on both knees, girl, and eat of dirt; you can't do this alone.

What is this tide sifting the sand at my feet, leaving me to follow? Don't wanna move. Can't bring myself to dance. Some God or Goddess took insult, rooted me to the ground. Leaves and branches grow more each day behind my eyes and obscure my view. Take my life, this tangled thicket. Prune me back to a green and glistening bud with care. With that perhaps this weary heart can breathe again, fearless, inhale God's fragrance of a riotous spring.

> *Speak to me of love, and the glory of devotion.*
> *Forgive my silly terror of the night.*
> *Elucidate the verse of psalms, hymns,*
> *Those where the child gives way to light.*

A Dream of Famine

i'm working hard *at my desk. I suddenly remember that I've forgotten to nurse my newborn. I reach into my desk drawer and remove a small container. I gently tap its surface until the baby slides into the palm of my hand. I am unsure how to feed my tiny, inch-long child, its skin pink and glistening as a rodent embryo. I nudge its lips with an eyedropper, but the stem is much too large.*

The skin on its head is slightly shriveled and its eyes are unseeing, mere hollowed indentations. Studying its limitations, I become increasingly anxious over having neglected its nourishment. Gradually, the child changes shape. I still attempt to feed what is now only a tiny pair of lips, a cup-shaped sucking mouth that fusses. I place the baby mouth like a cap on my nipple, where it begins to nurse.

As I sit with my breasts exposed, my black dress stripped down around my waist, a group of office workers crowd around to observe me. I feel a twinge of selfishness for what has now become a public moment of eroticism. A potent sense of guilt attempts to upbraid my reprehensible pleasure and, to my delight, it fails. When they finish nursing, I detach the sleepy lips and observe them. Now, no features are apparent, no child, and no lips. Lying in my palm is a simple, fleshy disc drained of meaning, a single cooked, buttery, orecchiette pasta shell, a small repast of delectable metaphor for me.

I

Writing, my hands go slack on the keyboard. My focus shatters and drops its petals collectively. As my skin begins to buzz, I get up with a rough push of my chair to make my fourth cup of herbed tea. Anxious, I wander around the kitchen and forage limited rewards of sweet or salty food.

I've worked all day to screw down three hundred words into wood. This book, these stories I'm trying to write, what are they to me, a way back home, a reckoning? I'm mapping the past and revisiting the cavernous realm of illness to learn what I can. Like a redeemed and transformed maid of myths, I turn back to study my own likeness in that of the dying Gorgon. Her metastasized snakes lie cold and quiet, but her eyes still have the power to turn me to stone.

I sit down at the desk again to face the region between my thoughts and the page. My sentences fall in and out of third-person singular, my only protection against the descriptive remembrance of illness. The crucial facts are still so recent, not yet tamed and deified by the ripening light of the past. I whine and shimmy up to beg at the lap of memory. Give it to me gentle, an eloquent phrase with which to saw at the knees of a moment, lest I blank you out, numb as an amnesiac, and erase for a lifetime the dark edge of divinity.

II

Love's arms are waiting, strong, resilient and delicious. Death casts no shadow on the eager smile in my lover's eyes. I feel myself succumbing. Will the visage of a tumor, real or unreal, snatch away this sweetness and trample on well-laid plans? Will I have the courage to love someone new? The briar and the berry of connectedness twine about my aspirations, a tortured garland. At dawn my heart wakes first, nervous and preachy as a spinster. "Love's a hazard. I wouldn't risk attachment in your shoes. Terribly risky!" I open my eyes and gaze at the calm, sleeping face of my lover. Harry appreciates that death might be found in any moment, here or on any street in town.

III

I put down the *Atlantic Monthly*, cover my face with my hands and weep. The premise of the article is that chemotherapy as a cure does little to no good. Most cancer patients recur and die according to the length of time it took to grow their original tumor. The chiseled words of the breast-cancer research doctor enter me like barbed hooks. I know it will take months to extract them all. Each negative statistic breeds a little self-propelled fear. They burrow their way into my psyche. There, under the thin skin of confidence, one honeycombed wound infects the next. Like foxtail burrs from a favorite sock worth saving, I'll pluck his findings from the glossy new pelt of my fragile hopes.

IV

After two years, a stray canister of film proves to contain photographs from Christmas 1994, the night I returned home from the stem-cell transplant. Shuffling through them, I find a picture of my brother and me, sitting with his arm around me on my sister's couch. In the close-up image of my own ravaged face, I see a person who has traveled in the company of Death.

The Christmas portrait conspires against me in memory, bringing back the shock, the yellow color and smell of illness. For a moment, gravity holds its breath and I have to brace my own body upright. My gaze focuses on my photographed eyes: speck of diamond rudely puncturing the pupil's black pool in the center of the iris. In those eyes, I recognize a last personification of my ill-at-ease self, a tainted vestigial presence that might somehow have the power to summon me back, betrayed by Orpheus.

V

On the second anniversary of my cancer surgery, Harry and I and the dogs return from a camp by a river northwest of us. The temperature has reached 105 in the shade. As we approach the gravel road into the ranch, we see the dramatic evidence of a fire.

I learn that the mountain house I have rented for fifteen years has been saved by a set of coincidences. A policeman took the scenic route. Seeing the smoke, he alerted volunteer crews, minutes after the grass fire began to spread. My brother spotted the smoke at my location on the mountain from miles away on the highway, and rushed there to help. One hundred and twenty firefighters, ten engines, two helicopters and various friends and relatives descended in our absence. The fire line is a few steps off the old flagstone patio.

The woods along the road to the house are a foot deep in ash where the path of the blaze has whooshed up the canyon. Rooted in cinder, black, smoking trees struggle to maintain their flow of sap. I wander around, stunned by the obvious intervention that has protected me. A deeper meaning emerges and supersedes consideration of the loss of my material world. Anxiety has driven me from every attempt to write the story of my bone-marrow transplant. All summer, I've been unable to court the imagery, the central metaphor of fire or chemotherapy as a Burning. When all the stories of the actual wildfire have been told, what happened when and where, the facts of the firefight seem like the highly choreographed inventions of a playwright. Are the real and metaphorical fires a grand coincidence or something more? Has the frustrated analogy lifted itself from the page, proclaimed itself a high sign that fascinates me with all its aspects?

It does not matter whether or not it is possible for metaphor or inspiration to manifest in reality. At this moment it seems possible, and the tandem events of real fire and metaphor is vastly useful. Mumbo jumbo or no, it's just the hook I need to hang on. Fact is stranger than fiction and the fire is a juncture that helps me forget my troubles.

I know that I will witness the hillside's recovery. I've been given an exquisitely illustrated daybook of regeneration for my year. Some trees will live and flourish; many will die. Extraordinary views have now been revealed and the sun freshens what were once dank corners. I know that unusual birds and insects will arrive to make use of this process of rebirth. Very possibly there will be rare wildflowers. Vitality will reemerge in its own time.

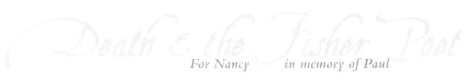

For Nancy   in memory of Paul

Dear friend, your voice on the phone is tragic. You tell me you have inoperable tumors in your lungs and other places. The knowledge of your cancer punctures me. It slides under my skin like a blunt needle threaded with the fiber of fond memories and the poignant regret of lost opportunities. Your news enters me and stitches a crude seam through my innards, blindly working its way through my muscle and tissue, the power in you allowing your news to be both fatal and optimistic, suturing as it cuts across the weathered prairie of my loving.

Harry and I bring you presents in the VA hospital. I start holding my breath when I see you hooked to tubes and medical equipment. Sitting up cross-legged on the bed, you take care of me and dispel our awkwardness with lighthearted jokes, witty commentary and little smiles.

Turning to include them, you introduce us to the four other men in your room, reciting their stories as though you'd known them for years. One has been a salmon fisherman like you. You ignore the implications of contrived fellowship between you, taking special care to include the loneliest in our conversation. You pass amongst them the basket of delicacies I've brought you, taking nothing for yourself. I leave you, shocked by your pallor and your courage. Mine has deserted me.

Each time we meet I see that Death sucks hard on the straw that drains your life. Each time we talk, the conversation is shorter than the last. You were very afraid of dying for a short time. Now you fear only how Death will come to you. In the end you are tired of homage and desire, as it should be, only your family around you. You leave us in autumn, jump off bravely and with humor into what you believe to be worms and Nothingness, leaving us the priceless benefit of your noble example. I bring sage leaves from the Sierras to scent your homemade casket. At the request of your wife and sons, I write a few words for your funeral that I hope will lessen the grief of those who loved you most.

Weeks have passed since your death, but your rejection of an afterlife of consciousness continues to trouble me. I speak to you in my thoughts but you do not answer, in dreams or otherwise. In your honor I hold a fiesta on Day of the Dead. I exhaust myself cooking an elaborate meal for friends who knew you. By celebrating, I hope to dispel my fears. You see, half dreaming, in my prayers before sleep, I have seen you falling, spinning in a universe of stars, your face a stark mask lit with transformative flames.

For the fiesta, I decorate a large altar and place your picture there. I surround it with gifts: a cigarette of your liking and demise, special rocks and shells you've given me, a pen and scrap of paper for your poems, a small bird's nest with eggs. Amidst the magenta crowns of giant cockscomb flowers, fruited tangerine branches and marigolds sit squat bottles of beer, a basket of small golden lady apples, colored plates stacked with sugared discs of dark chocolate, garlands of tiny red peppers.

In the midst of all of this you smile at me from a favorite color photograph splintered with age. Energetic, elbows bent forward on your knees, you grin and laugh. Here, you finally have something to say. Your special goodbye phrase, "You have a good dream tonight, OK?"

Mortal Again

My wings are long dry, loyal reader. Two years have passed. When frightening memories overtake me, I privately cower in post-traumatic stress. I've spent too much time measuring the urgency of each day and imagining the worst against a backdrop of every bright hope. The daily routine of my job encroaches on contemplative pursuits, as part-time hours become full-time, plus a long commute. My wish for solitude and the creative process is replaced with financial concerns and the welcoming of job promotion and mounting responsibilities. My scattered attempts at meditation and prayer are again plagued with unexpectedly violent imagery. My sense of surrender to sources larger than my life alternately falters and blossoms with humility and heat. Through all of this, intimate or remote, the compassionate presence of the Virgin Mother remains a touchstone of every day.

The new metal of myself emerges in significant ways with actions of a more confident self. I choose urgency over stillness, flush paychecks over poverty, but still attempt to "have it all." In the midnight kingdom of after-hours, I'm a Midas of minutes, demanding perfection and creative manifestation from a mighty, chugging train of days. Each one could prove my last before some terrifying rediscovery. I am a hopeless creature of habit and the familiar grooves of my psychology embrace the familiarity of old myths and behaviors. Accomplishments are the measure of life well lived. Hard work equals goodness. Avoiding confrontation is commensurate with security. Love others more than yourself. A terrible tension exists between this habitual state of ethics and a new desire to expand a birth of consciousness leading me to acceptance rather than drive, the power of simplicity rather than ambition, humility and anonymous altruism opposed to proven and glorified performance, but, most important of all, quiet and loving self-reverence put forth before the needs of others.

Will I fail the great opportunity of new life and belief in an abundant and benevolent universe; will I stay mired in old, unhealthy ways? Is true change only a mechanism of disaster? A sibling asks, "Why do you make such a big deal of it all, anyway? Just enjoy yourself now that you're well." What does the Virgin say? "Be true to yourself. Love and care for the ones you're with. Quiet yourself and your truest center will unfold. Never lie about your feelings or cheat yourself of honesty. Stay unattached to outcome."

Still, I repeatedly analyze my fears; I question my motives and my destiny. I endure protracted stalls in my ability to write, writing being the creative process I now identify with survival. The necessary stamina to inhabit the spiritual past and describe the power of illness is often absent. I find myself stumbling from one day into the next, fatigued by my motivation to use what time I have. I ask myself, if I keep writing these letters to my disease, heaven knows what might rise from the past. Will fear overtake me? What am I dancing with? Who is that faintly calling?

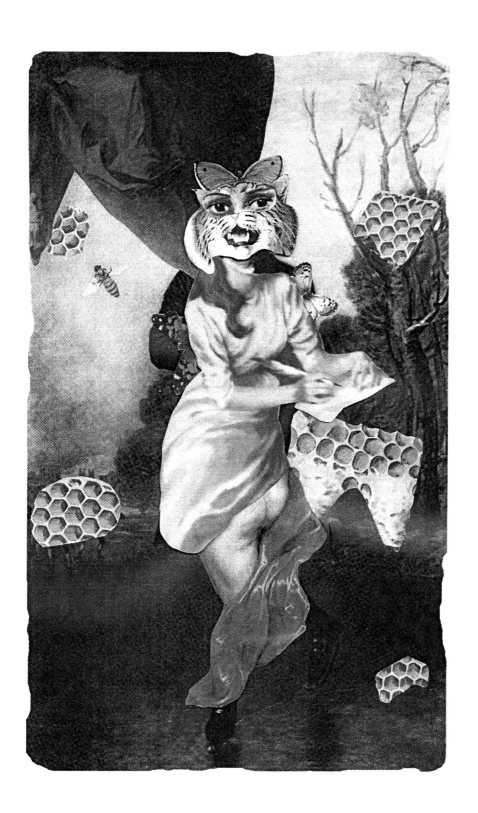

I'm
haunted by the specter of a new tumor. It has
its shadowy way with me, informs and taunts my psyche. Fear
is its companion. They lope behind me or yap together in the periphery
and herd me with their heavy and gangly paws. My instinct has me run-
ning, frantic, toward the trap of intangible safety. My uncombed hair gives
me away. Hidden inside is a desire to bleat and froth in wide-eyed
frenzy, afraid to glance back and write it, for fear of falling
on treacherous ground.

The hours

spent in the genesis of these sentences are hours that I've turned 'round to face fear. I write with a knife between my teeth and these lettered keys are my weapons in both hands. Each of my stories is a dance within a battle of invisible forces, a graceful turn and a twist, a thrusting gyration and momentary brace against the blows of cellular circumstance.

These words will be what survive me. Much time has passed since I began. Writing, I revisit a dark passage, the tale of a little life, strug-gling to be reborn. My yearning for divine presence fortifies me. I know that in vanquishing fear, I'll return again to the nurturing arms of a Mother God whose love medicine is my fortune to claim.

VIII. THE FRUIT OF ASHES

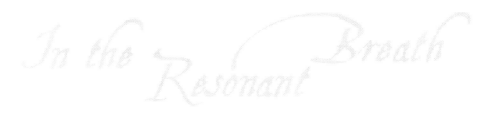

The longer I maintain good health, the more dramatic my fear of death becomes. The weeks before my biannual exam, my anxiety and that of family and friends solidifies. The relief we feel after the exam is profound. Yet for me, within months of verifying the absence of disease, doubt creeps in again. My oncologist tells me that compared to most, this is atypical, and a friend describes my state of mind as death-row psychology. Maybe it's the little happy pills that are missing? The drug protocol of antidepressants for cancer patients is something I'm reluctant to accept, though it could neutralize the aftermath of feeling and calm my dread.

After a tearful conversation, my oncologist lingers with me, genuinely concerned for my state of mind. He asks me, why are you so hard on yourself? Why do you have to chart the territory of your own fear? In HMO appointment intervals, it's difficult to explain to him all that is in my mind. The clinical environment intimidates me and my motives for avoiding antidepressants are so complex personally and creatively that I decide against attempting to explain. Instead, I seek to validate myself by questioning him. Don't you think, after what I've been through, I have a right to feel sad and angry? Don't you think my emotions are appropriate to reconciling the physiological turmoil of my body caused by the blunt revisions of the chemical menopause?

I am attaining the private world of my womanhood through a ritualized process of facing mortality. This process brings art and meaning to my life. If fearing an early death is what generates creative renewal, so be it. I don't want to circumvent any of it. It's true, I want out of the psychological roulette I play, this game of *How long before I die?* But would antidepressants vaporize the muse and make all these questions and self-serious myth making seem unnecessary, even ridiculous? Am I a prude or a snob, listening to a little voice that says, "Pills? It's not like you to choose the easy route"? Is the acknowledgement of the dark side worth the mental anguish of unadulterated reality, and does this moment-by-moment architecture of renewal hold life's highest purpose?

After listening to me thoughtfully and respectfully, my oncologist lovingly sends me home with sample packets of Zoloft. They find a resting place in a kitchen cupboard, where I forget them and the advantage or disadvantage of their potency finally expires.

I placed my trust in you and chose to do what you asked of me. If you had risked warning me of every result would I have turned from your best advice? Besieged by changes of every type, doubting my choices in the aftermath of treatment is a part of our bond as patient and physician. How can I articulate for you that my process of reckoning inhabits the very heart of my survival like an orchestrated theme, my fears numbered beats in a rhythmic score of inspiration? I'm singing into being the song of my "Death Reality." I want to live in a world where each of the greatest composers puts to music the words "I will die" and every citizen has time to listen and respond.

I go back to telling myself that disease or not, you could die anytime. You don't control the scheduling of your death, so stop worrying and hurrying. Enjoy life; take joyful pleasure in each day you have.

Gratefully consider millions of other people in the world who will never be offered, much less afford, the medicine you've had the benefit of. I remind myself that life is more than the roles I have always played. I have everything I need. What I need is love, and love is all around me. In the midst of chronic anxiety, what I desire most is another intoxicating glimpse of divine presence embodied in the transition from disease to health.

I

LOMA'S SPRING RETREAT

Meditating in a circle with others, I do my best to banish expectation; still, my stealth mind sorts through its sack of tricks. My thoughts are busy bees hoping to alight on the perfectly opened flower of spiritual sensation.

Finally, my inner eye catches view of a brightly lit billboard. In a script of red letters it reads, "Afraid to discover what waits in silence?" I accept this challenge and see myself dodge under the sign, up an unlit street, escaping into stillness. I leave my stupefied mind, like a suspended matrix, transfixed by the measure of its own desires.

For a long while, I do nothing but breathe. At some point, I find a boyish version of myself walking in the underworld of a waking dream. I converse intimately with a vibrant persona, a long-haired embodiment of Intuition, dressed in flowing garments. She leads me by the hand along a lush, cavernous riverbank, cooled by a massive outcropping of hanging rock. The spare words of the muse ring like chimes against the echoing stone. Abruptly, she stops, and, turning, forcefully slaps my face with the front, then the back of her hand. She grips my upper arms and, shaking them, searches my eyes with her own. My shoulders go limp and she bears my weight.

Vast lettered essays of loopy hieroglyph litter the grassy bank and entangle our feet. At the sound of her slap, the letters leap to attention at our ankles and transform themselves into fragile flowers. I stand in a green meadow where they grow. I lift my gaze and in response, grass germinates and spreads from where I stand into an imagined distance. I breathe in fresh air and, bending back my head, realize that I am once again with others beneath sky above ground.

II

During meditation, my body is circled with spinning bands of colored aura. Sparks and pigment-saturated chunks of light fly off. I go inside my bloodstream and in miniature board a tiny boat. With an eye out for tumors, I sail along my arteries in a rush of red churning rapids. In the vast interior of the bloodstream, I moor my craft on a spit of bone and, squatting on haunches, build a fire. Lightly running along the shoreline toward me, my father and brothers approach. At the sight of them, waves of love wash through me.

III

I'm instructed to breathe rapidly for forty-five minutes. Questions and doubts swarm through my mind. Could I lose my breath or my control over everything? On a card I write, "I have nothing to fear." Within five minutes of rapid breathing, energy is coursing through my torso, arms and legs. Time passes very quickly. Panting, my limbs begin to vibrate and my arms rise upward of their own volition. My lips contract to form a hard white serrated circle through which a sound emerges at long intervals, a spontaneous om, independent of my breathing.

At the summit of this crazy energy an unexpected presence emerges. The Virgin hovers over me once more. My elevated hands are perfectly positioned to caress her brown face, smiling eyes bordered by her starry veil. Lightning rods of joy pierce my chest and abdomen. The ceiling fills with a kaleidoscope image of a thousand veiled Goddesses, eating the world then birthing it whole. Flames encircle this geometric universe where jewel colors of orange and violet pulsate in a tapestry of glory.

The Virgin's body levitates upward, pushes through the roof, and expands into the glittering night sky. Her chest and upper belly vanish to form a circular portal. I stand with my hands pressed flat against its sides and my feet braced firmly. In zero gravity, I stand balanced in her body and float with her amidst the black spaces between stars. I am the key in the keyhole of her heart center. Through it pass galaxies of planets and stars.

Only one message, in her unmistakable voice, permeates my being. "Live in me and none of your questions will matter. Give yourself to me and the rest, all your concerns, will be of no consequence."

One last question attempts to lay brick in my busy mind. "When will I die?"

"Die in me and live."

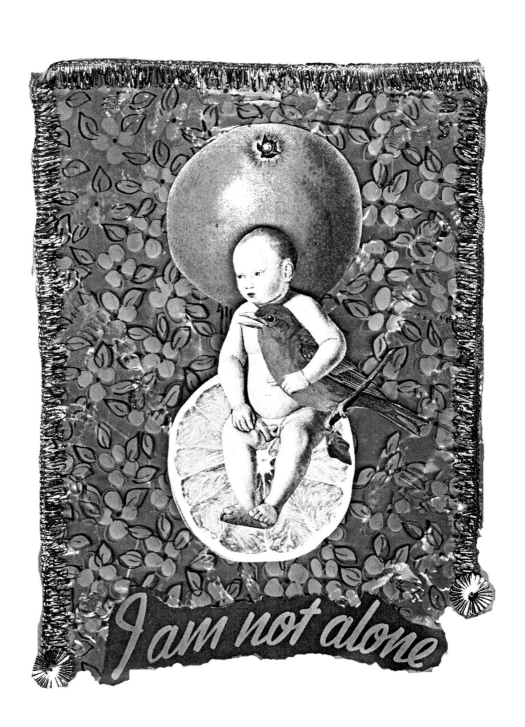

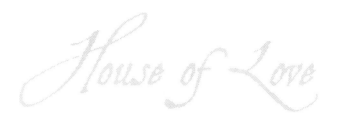

House of Love

We stoke the coals of desire in a stony hearth
Through windows we learn of the soul
Inside this roof of realized flesh and foundation of bone
Our heart, a fathomless well
Fed by an unseen aquifer of spirit
Mysterious to us.

Inside this house of love is where I want to be.
To live!
Inside this house, a fragrant bough,
I rest in you, oh my beloved.

Once again, waltzing paper skeletons, wreaths of crab apples, man-darins and marigolds decorate the mantle above a kindled fire. Four celebration altars are ablaze with candlelight to which both public and private offerings have been made. Lanterns and torches lead to the shrine in the garden. The Virgin's image resides here anew, together with clusters of flower petals, floating on water and lit by the red and blue glass of votive candles. Guadalupe's sad smile is reflected in the tiny pool.

The creatures of the woods listen to the sound of fifty women laughing, their revelry floating on the air of autumn twilight. We delight in each other's stories, drink wine, eat and dance. Late into the night, we keep each other quiet company by the patio fire. All of us are hungry for meaning and the luxury of tranquil reflection, diverse female friends brought together to celebrate the feminine in its many characters and forms. My recovery gives my friends hope as their affection gives sweetness and purpose to my life.

My mother is amongst the revelers, wearing flowers in her hair. Even in her seventies, she is often the first to dance at any party. I learned the importance of ritual and Magic Realism by her example and long reliance on the properties of imagination and faith. After striving at an early age to separate from her and claim my own iden-tity, I discover the shared experience of breast cancer has deepened the intimacy between us. I not only appreciate but understand now her courageousness as a young mother facing the loss her death would mean to five young children.

She sustained herself through the disfigurement of radical mastectomy, the lack of medical finesse and the social taboo of the fifties, moving forward to raise her children alone in her forties and in the process achieving financial independence and professional recognition without a recurrence of disease. I recall no incidence in our life together where my mother ever complained of her misfortune. Breast cancer was only a topic in regards to the rules of prevention she took pains to instill in my sister and me or the problem of bathing suits, the expense of a new prosthesis or style restrictions of necklines. Practical matters were devoid of self-pity and infused, more often than not, with humor. Her life story can easily be viewed as one destructive blow after another by which she refuses to be categorized. An intensely creative person, she prefers the model of noble heroism that she has taught so wisely and so artfully, encouraging us to shine brightly and do the best we can.

The closest of my female friends are also in my company tonight, those who lit the course of my life-changing descent and visited me with devotion of thought and caring. I am surrounded by a constellation of individuals to be guided by, who provide a repository of loving qualities the memory of which lives forever inside me. The charitable healing of Janet's hands, Jill's daily cards, Mary's fearlessness, Maureen's courage and Dinah's returning with wit and energy. Kimberly's art, Gretchen's maternal concern, Amy's determined alliance, Jeani's unconditional love, Julie, compassionate, intelligent mother.

Anita to the rescue, Loma opening new worlds and Tej and Maria left to lovingly deal with the anxious concern of my brothers. All my many unnamed friends whose letters, conversation and acts of loving-kindness make life worth celebrating.

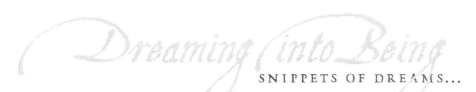
Messages of resolution from an inner script begin to surface in metaphorical dreams. These dreams are distilled parables of my journey, vivid trailers from the live cinema of my psyche. Interacting with mythic themes and guides, I deconstruct, in dreams, the aftermath of my transformative process, catastrophe to completion. In my unconscious, I view the wreckage, meet with allies and heal my wounds.

I

...steering a jeep, *I drive through the winding streets of a remote village, which people have abandoned. Paved with weathered cobblestones and crumbling brick, the streets are littered with the fresh, unmolested carcasses of exotic animals. Against curbs and doorways I see a woolly ox, giraffe, ostrich, bears and gazelle. On a corner, we find Kandinsky's blue horse slumped in an alcove. I am told the animals died here, after the sail of the ark...*

II

i swim, tirelessly, *in an ocean of lapis-colored seawater. No land is in sight. Alongside me swims a fluorescent green serpent, lit like neon. Seven feet long and a foot wide, his friendly face is marvelously alert as he lifts his*

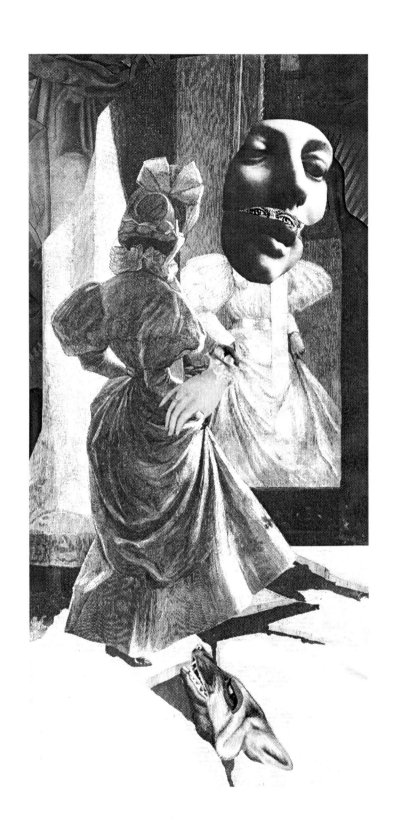

head and upper body to face me. I embrace him and, facing one another, we move in tandem through the surge.

As I swim excitedly, enraptured to shore, another swimmer appears in the shallower water. He announces that the snake is dead. As I pull my companion from the receding wave, I see that what he says is true. The serpent is now emptied and flat, a faded sheet of greenish scales that lifts in the breeze like a tattered kite. The swimmer cautions me that the husk of skin may harbor deadly poisons, retained long after shedding.

in my dream *I attend a festive party, hosted by my mother. My father sings light opera to applause. As guests drift about, I find myself distracted by the beauty of a large bowl of ripe persimmons.*

I show my friends, Amy and Maureen, a Life *magazine photograph of a woman swimming underwater. She purls with the current amongst fish of all kinds, large and small, sharks and salmon. She is fully clothed in sealskin and has webbed feet, and a knapsack is lashed to her back. Her black hair, parted down the middle, slicks to her forehead as she propels herself through the swells, arms at her side, hair floating, flippers kicking, tiny bubbles rising.*

Later, I see her here, at the party, but she doesn't engage me. I watch her from a distance as she moves about and then stands, dripping in a doorway. She carries a slender harpoon loosely balanced in one hand. She is, I know, highly educated, a medicine woman who breathes with gills. No one else in the room seems to notice her.

She turns toward me, staring, and her penetrating eyes draw us both to a farther place. I find myself holding the hand of my grandmother who died, years ago, at the age of one hundred. Much older now, wrinkles track her face in a spidery maze. Her shrunken body sits upright, surrounded by heavy gray blankets, and her eyes are brimming with tears. She wears no shoes and her childlike feet are worn with exposure.

Haltingly, she tells me that she regrets not having been more loving in life. Rocking back and forth, her tear-filled eyes are lit with a bright spark beneath fallen lids. Again and again, she grips my arm, repeating, "If only I'd looked at you, all of you in the eyes and told you how I loved you. I loved you."

IV

i lie on *the ground bleeding in a crossroad surrounded by open fields, fenced by distant trees. I sprawl there in a dirty brown robe, reduced to rags. The amount of blood pooling around me suggests that I've suffered a mortal wound. An elderly couple stands over me, their good shoes stained with bloody dirt. He, a professor, and his female counterpart, a teacher, are German intellectuals, perhaps ancestors. Kindly, they chastise me for losing heart. With heavy accents they admonish me, "Look at you. You must not give up. You must try harder." I grip my stomach; blood pulses from between my hands.*

They lower a tin plate full of beans and shredded meat and encourage me to feed myself. Propped on one arm, I do my best to move the spoon to my mouth. A group of children approaches us. A little girl steps toward me and announces, "I'm hungry." She asks that I carry her home. Lifting her to my shoulders, I straighten and stand. In the distance, I view a long windbreak of outlying trees. I know that when I reach them, I will have reentered the world.

My living room is crowded with guests chatting and visiting. In one corner, I reason with a depressed friend on the phone. Making conversation, I tell him, "Look at it this way: at least you haven't been stabbed." I'm wearing a pink, frilly party dress, which blood has soaked through from my abdomen. Smeared and drying, it cakes to the surface of its rosy sateen. Beneath my clothes the wound still oozes and drips. Abruptly, a young artist in a beret approaches me with his palette. Swiftly, he dips his brush and begins to paint the front of my dress, mixing his pigment with my blood.

I cruise through the streets of a dangerous neighborhood. With my hands I apply pressure to the aching slice under my shirt. I consider going into a real-estate office to complete the purchase of property, but resist. The stress could activate the return of bleeding, reveal my injuries to the agent and jeopardize the contract.

In pouring rain, I walk down a rutted, gravel road beneath my house in the woods. Again, in a ragged brown robe with a cowl and hood, I carry a staff and bundle of sticks cut from long branches. Powerful rivulets of water course down the culverts and across the gravel. I have come to repair a washout.

On the road, I meet a group of medieval women carrying babies. Numerous small children with ruddy cheeks and wet wool leggings trail behind them. Traveling on foot, food and dry kindling are bundled in the women's backpacks and in the folds of their long skirts. They grow nervous at the sight of me, but I put them at ease over our encounter by playfully admiring their offspring. As we talk, our breath fogs the air until, smiling, they continue on their journey. I inhale the spice of wet evergreen and feel ecstatically at one with the world. I decide against damming the flooding water to let nature take its course.

Walking back up the road, I think to check my wound. Exposing a patch of white skin to the rain, I finger all that remains of it: a thin and ropy line. As I pinch my flesh, it squeezes open like a bloodless paper cut, still deep, but somehow closed, healed, a perfectly clean and painless vestibule. I'm satisfied by what I see. By the side of the road I find several large chunks of glistening black obsidian, wet with rain. I hurry to show Harry what I've found.

FORTY-FIFTH BIRTHDAY, AUGUST 8, 1999

Early-morning mist drops a beaded cloak across the tops of woodland trees, arousing fragrant oils. The conical body of a distant knoll ascends from a low fog settled between steep sides of the canyon stretching beneath me. Its feet in billowy clouds, the knoll magically floats, a rock-covered island peaked with firs, in a sky sea, of gray and pearl horizon.

Near me, a flock of tiny yellow finches arrive from the south. They crowd the glossy leaves of the orange tree, from which a few aging juice-filled fruits still linger. Their fluttering wings beat the moist air as they lightly hop from slender branches. Bruising blossoms and fruit, they fan the faint yet pungent cologne of citrus to where I sit at the open window.

In the baked and bay-scented woods of August, the buzzing chirp of finch song ignites an energetic current of sound that rises and electrifies the moistened air. Within this indecipherable doctrine of birdsong and morning mist, a coded signal presents itself to me; a diminutive tributary of the Mother's radiance finds me and fills me with joy. Her message, like her love, a riddle of abundance...

Blossom scent on air perfume...the taste of one fruit imagines an orchard.
In my ear, consecrated harmonies of field song...
The sight of one beloved face forgives the sins of failed humanity.
Both riddle & answer at the end...all knowing STILL a question.
Love lives in eyes and hands, sleeps and riots in the heart...
Faith keeps like cold ground given life by a seasonal sun.

When I learned of my ten cancerous lymph nodes, I practiced letting go of everything I loved. That way, it would be easier to say goodbye when I died young. Instead I thrive, and struggle to fully reattach to life again. Allow relationships to deepen despite the odds that were once so against me. Community and hope, not detachment, has been the greater lesson.

I long for intimacy with the Virgin. The aura of Divine Feminine, that descends, comforts and instructs in the art of surrender; that deeply private grace that surrounds and envelops when most in need. But, she vanishes at the slightest distraction of earthy delights, love and success in living, of which I have a greater share. I mourn the slow and incremental loss of acute spiritual awareness. But my belief in divine nature sustains me, I know that I am not alone. Along with the support of those that love me, I defy a cynical culture and trust my body as it is, an aging temple honoring the desires of the lyrical nucleus intuitively articulated to the mind.

A potentially terminal illness provides a simple life strategy, reliance on great themes. Accept what is given moment by moment, abandon the status quo and speak your truth. Take what you have and make it beautiful; life is almost never as it seems. As I prepared for publication, rereading my manuscript several times, the memory of a poem surfaced, written down years ago from a dream about Jonah and the whale.

Oh mighty fish all black and shining that rules my mind and leaves me pining, grant a wish or take me under lost to icy corridors of slumber...

The thought of it persisted until I searched through old journals to rediscover that 1984 was the year I had written it, the calendar period my oncologist identified as the origin of my tumor in time. As I reread the words of the poem twenty years later, I recognized cipher encrypted in the metaphors, the mysterious communiqué of cells and psyche.

If you love me read my mind, discover the secret none can find...

Foretelling that, ransomed by disease, I would be delivered from isolation in the context of myth, evicted onto the shores of my own life holding in my body the "secret none can (yet) find."

A ship, a crew, a captain so handsome, all unknowing of my ransom...

There, by use of "fire and wit" burn away perceptions that have bound me.

Whilst I like Jonah by fire and wit, crowd the dark, the eternal myth...
I go aground on that desolate beach, and the coal of myself is all that I keep.

Take only the "coal of myself" to keep, those magnificent, cinder-cells wrought of chemotherapy and bravely regenerating in marrow.

There is a young child I hold onto inside myself. She is essential, more important than happiness or power. I try never to let loose of her hand, though distracted again and again. She needs my affectionate care, the light of my adoring gaze. In remembering the needs of her body I am one with myself. Born of fire, she is the Mother's daughter, moving my feet in dance.

Epiphany

To you...oh Mother of black hair
Mother of dusty feet
For you... Divine Mother of the sad smile
Mother of the sensuous heart
Of you...fierce procreator
Mother of flesh-filled teeth
In you Mother...the grace of the verdant heart
Fresh with childlike pleasure
Through you...oh Mother of pitiless strength
Mother of untapped resource
Because of you...Mother of disastrous surrender
Mother of wings
Mother of wet ground
Mother of the moments between moments
Mother of rustling leaves and shifting breezes
Send your earth messenger
Original Virgin, harbinger, Mother of mysterious blood Find
my scent
on dry
leaves

SPECIAL ACKNOWLEDGEMENT AND THANKS

To my mother Jane, a writer with heart, who listens and encourages with love. To the physicians and healers who came to my aide so skillfully and lovingly: Dr Robert Hall, Dr. Daniel Mirda, Dr. John Dermody, Dr. Leland Raymond, Nancy Tulley and Janet Blum. In acknowledgement of love and inspiration, to Jim Harrison for his friendship and letters that so sustained me, my cousin Paule Anglim for her support and elegance of thought and Nancy Garden, guardian of culture who never fails to inspire. Editor Sheryl Fullerton, who early on encouraged the literary voice and Theresa Whitehill, of Colored Horse Studios, for her superb design work, perseverance and collaborative spirit. In dedication to Harry, with me in the dark places of a doubtful night and still the cheerful morn.

The Art of Surrender
was typeset in Bembo, with
Aquiline Chapter Titling, and Hadriano Heads

DESIGN AND PRODUCTION
Colored Horse Studios, Ukiah, California
www.coloredhorse.com

PRE-PRESS & SCANNING ASSISTANCE
Brendan Smith

COPY EDITING
Julia Bloch

PROOFREADING
Cheryl Maslin

BECCA SMITH

GLANCING ORPHEUS PRESS

ACORN BANK, MIDDLETOWN, CALIFORNIA

Signed copies available by contacting the author
bsmith@oberondesign.com
www.theartofsurrender.com

Printed in the United States
106356LV00006B/19/A

9 781589 613874